SO-BEB-054

ECSI **Emergency Care** and **Safety Institute**

Preventing Infectious Diseases

Fifth Edition

Jeffrey Lindsey, PhD
Medical Writer

Benjamin Gulli, MD
Medical Editor

Jon R. Krohmer, MD, FACEP
Medical Editor

American College of
Emergency Physicians®

ADVANCING EMERGENCY CARE

JONES AND BARTLETT PUBLISHERS

Sudbury, Massachusetts

BOSTON   TORONTO   LONDON   SINGAPORE

Jones and Bartlett Publishers

World Headquarters
40 Tall Pine Drive
Sudbury, MA 01776
info@jbpub.com
www.ECSInstitute.org

Jones and Bartlett Publishers Canada
6339 Ormindale Way
Mississauga, Ontario L5V 1J2
Canada

Jones and Bartlett Publishers International
Barb House, Barb Mews
London W6 7PA
United Kingdom

Jones and Bartlett's books and products are available through most bookstores and online booksellers. To contact Jones and Bartlett Publishers directly, call 800-832-0034, fax 978-443-8000, or visit our website www.jbpub.com.

Substantial discounts on bulk quantities of Jones and Bartlett's publications are available to corporations, professional associations, and other qualified organizations. For details and specific discount information, contact the special sales department at Jones and Bartlett via the above contact information or send an email to specialsales@jbpub.com.

AAOS
AMERICAN ACADEMY OF
ORTHOPAEDIC SURGEONS

Editorial Credits
Chief Education Officer: Mark W. Wieting
Director, Department of Publications: Marilyn L. Fox, PhD
Managing Editor: Barbara A. Scotese

Board of Directors 2006
Richard F. Kyle, MD, President
James H. Beaty, MD
E. Anthony Rankin, MD
William L. Healy, MD
Gordon M. Aamoth, MD
Leslie L. Altick
Dwight W. Burney, III, MD
John T. Gill, MD
Joseph C. McCarthy, MD
Norman Otsuka, MD
Andrew N. Pollak, MD
Matthew S. Shapiro, MD
James P. Tasto, MD
Kristy Weber, MD
Stuart L. Weinstein, MD
Ken Yamaguchi, MD
Karen L. Hackett, FACHE, CAE (Ex-Officio)

Production Credits
Chief Executive Officer: Clayton Jones
Chief Operating Officer: Donald W. Jones, Jr.
President, Higher Education and Professional Publishing: Robert W. Holland, Jr.
V.P., Sales and Marketing: William J. Kane
V.P., Production and Design: Anne Spencer
V.P., Manufacturing and Inventory Control: Therese Connell
Publisher: Lawrence D. Newell
Publisher, Public Safety: Kimberly Brophy
Acquisitions Editor: Christine Emerton

Production Supervisor: Jenny L. Corriveau
Photo Research Manager/Photographer: Kimberly Potvin
Director of Marketing: Alisha Weisman
Interior Design: Anne Spencer
Cover Design: Kristin E. Ohlin
Cover Image: © LiquidLibrary
Composition: Shepherd, Inc.
Text Printing and Binding: Courier Kendallville
Cover Printing: Courier Kendallville

Copyright © 2008 by Jones and Bartlett Publishers, Inc.

All rights reserved. No part of the material protected by this copyright notice may be reproduced or utilized in any form, electronic or mechanical, including photocopying, recording, or by any information storage and retrieval system, without written permission from the copyright owner.

The procedures in this book are based on the most current recommendations of responsible medical sources. The American Academy of Orthopaedic Surgeons and the Publisher, however, make no guarantee as to, and assume no responsibility for, the correctness, sufficiency, or completeness of such information or recommendations. Other or additional safety measures may be required under particular circumstances.

Reviewed by the American College of Emergency Physicians
The American College of Emergency Physicians (ACEP) makes every effort to ensure that its product and program reviewers are knowledgeable content experts and recognized authorities in their fields. Readers are nevertheless advised that the statements and opinions expressed in this publication are provided as guidelines and should not be construed as College policy unless specifically referred to as such. The College disclaims any liability or responsibility for the consequences of any actions taken in reliance on those statements or opinions. The materials contained herein are not intended to establish policy, procedure, or a standard of care. To contact ACEP write to: PO Box 619911, Dallas, TX 75261-9911; call toll-free 800-798-1822, touch 6, or 972-550-0911.

Library of Congress Cataloging-in-Publication Data
Lindsey, Jeffrey, 1963–
 Preventing infectious disease / Jeffrey Lindsey.—5th ed.
  p. cm.
 Rev. ed. of: Preventing infectious diseases / Benjamin Gulli, editor; American Academy of Orthopaedic Surgeons. 4th rev. ed. © 2005.
 ISBN-13: 978-0-7637-4990-3 (pbk.)
 ISBN-10: 0-7637-4990-7 (pbk.)
 1. Bloodborne infections—Prevention. I. Title.
 RA642.B56T48 2007
 614.4'4—dc22
 6048   2006102063

Additional photographic and illustration credits appear on page 101, which constitutes a continuation of the copyright page.

Printed in the United States of America
11 10 09 08 07   10 9 8 7 6 5 4 3 2 1

contents

welcome

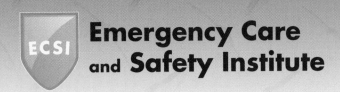

Emergency Care and Safety Institute

Welcome to the Emergency Care and Safety Institute

Welcome to the Emergency Care and Safety Institute (ECSI), brought to you by the American Academy of Orthopaedic Surgeons (AAOS) and the American College of Emergency Physicians (ACEP).

The ECSI is an educational organization created for the purpose of delivering the highest quality training to laypersons and professionals in the areas of First Aid, CPR, AED, Bloodborne Pathogens, and related safety and health fields.

Two of the most respected names in injury, illness, and emergency medical care—the AAOS and the ACEP—have approved the content in our training materials.

AAOS
AMERICAN ACADEMY OF
ORTHOPAEDIC SURGEONS

About the AAOS

The AAOS provides education and practice management services for orthopaedic surgeons and allied health professionals. The AAOS also serves as an advocate for improved patient care and informs the public about the science of orthopaedics. Founded in 1933, the not-for-profit AAOS has grown from a small organization serving less than 500 members to the world's largest medical association of musculoskeletal specialists. The AAOS now serves about 24,000 members internationally.

American College of Emergency Physicians®
About ACEP

ACEP was founded in 1968 and is the world's oldest and largest emergency medicine specialty organization. Today it represents more than 22,000 members and is the emergency medicine specialty society recognized as the acknowledged leader in emergency medicine.

ECSI Course Catalog

Individuals seeking training in ECSI subjects can choose from among various online and offline course offerings. The following courses are available through the ECSI:

First Aid, CPR, and AED Standard

CPR and AED

Professional Rescuer CPR

First Aid

Wilderness First Aid

Bloodborne Pathogens

First Responder

First Aid and CPR Online

First Aid Online

Adult CPR Online

Adult and Pediatric CPR Online

Professional Rescuer CPR Online

AED Online

Adult CPR and AED Online

Bloodborne Pathogens Online

The ECSI offers a wide range of textbooks, instructor and student support materials, and interactive technology, including online courses. Every ECSI textbook is the center of an integrated teaching and learning system that offers instructor, student, and technology resources to better support instructors and prepare students. The instructor supplements provide practical hands-on, time-saving tools like PowerPoint presentations, DVDs, and web-based distance learning resources. The student supplements are designed to help students retain the most important information and to assist them in preparing for exams. And, a key component to the teaching and learning systems are technology resources that provide interactive exercises and simulations to help students become great emergency responders.

Documents attesting to the ECSI's recognitions of satisfactory course completion will be issued to those who successfully meet the course objectives and criteria for passing the course. Written acknowledgement of a participant's successful course completion is provided in the form of a Course Completion Card, issued by the ECSI.

Visit www.ECSInstitute.org today!

resource preview

This textbook is the center of the bloodborne pathogens program with features that will reinforce and expand on the essential information.

Features include:

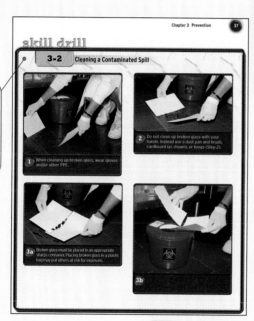

Skill Drills
Provide step-by-step explanations and visual summaries of important skills.

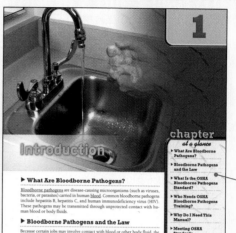

Chapter at a Glance
Guides students through the topics in that chapter.

Caution Boxes
Emphasize crucial actions that students should or should not take when the possibility of contact with a bloodborne pathogen exists.

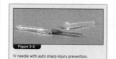

Figure 3-2

IV needle with auto sharp injury prevention.

Figure 3-3

Needleless system.

resource preview

FYI Boxes
Include valuable information related to bloodborne pathogens and prevention strategies.

Reproduced page — Chapter 2 Bloodborne Pathogens — 13

If you are exposed to bloodborne pathogens, a confidential medical evaluation is to be made *immediately* available to you, the injured employee. The word *immediately* is used in the standard to emphasize the importance of prompt medical evaluation and prophylaxis. An exact time cannot be stated because the time limit on the effectiveness of postexposure prophylactic measures does vary depending on the infection of concern.

Medical evaluation must be confidential and protect your identity and test results.

FYI

Activities Associated With Sharps Injuries

Needlestick and other sharps injuries are primarily associated with the following activities: disposing needles; administering injections; drawing blood, including the use of glass capillary tubes; recapping needles; and handling trash and dirty linens.

FYI

Blood Testing Results

Employers do not have a specific right to know the actual results of the source individual's blood testing, but they must ensure that the information is provided to the evaluating health care professional.

If you go for a medical evaluation, the following information will be made available to the health professional:

1. A copy of the OSHA guidelines section 1910.1030. This is the OSHA standard that dictates the requirement for all aspects of bloodborne pathogens and infectious diseases. The OSHA standard provides the necessary procedures for the medical evaluation.
2. A description of how the incident occurred as it relates to your employment
3. The results of the source individual's testing (if available)
4. All medical records that are relevant for your proper treatment (if treatment is necessary),

including a copy of your hepatitis B vaccination status with the dates of all the hepatitis B vaccinations and any medical records relative to your ability to receive the vaccination

You and your employer should expect that current Centers for Disease Control (CDC) guidelines will be used to guide postexposure prophylaxis and treatment.

It is the employer's responsibility to ensure that your medical records are kept confidential. Your records cannot be disclosed without your express written consent to any person within or outside the workplace, except as required by law. Your employer will have a copy of the health care provider's written opinion regarding the incident.

During consultation with the health professional, decisions will be made about the need for hepatitis B vaccination, and laboratory tests and information will be provided about available postexposure prophylaxis and treatments.

The health care professional will discuss the laboratory test results with you. A plan will be created that identifies any necessary follow-up or treatments, including initiation of hepatitis B immunization, if hepatitis B vaccine is indicated. Any postexposure treatments and follow-up plans should be in accordance with the current CDC guidelines.

▶ Reporting Requirements

What Is an Occupational Exposure Incident?

An occupational exposure incident occurs if you are in a work situation and come in contact with blood or OPIM.

For OSHA 2000 record-keeping purposes, an occupational bloodborne pathogens exposure incident (such as a needlestick, laceration, or splash) is classified as an injury because it is usually the result of an instantaneous event or exposure (**Figure 2.5**).

After an occupational exposure to blood or OPIM has occurred, the employee's name and job classification are listed on the OSHA 2000 log. The job classification should be reviewed, and a determination should be made as to which employees, if any, in that classification should now be covered under the standard.

Reproduced page — Chapter 2 Bloodborne Pathogens — 15

The California OSHA also requires the following:
- Identifying the body part involved in the exposure incident
- The engineering controls in use at the time if the sharp had engineered sharps injury protection
- Whether the protective mechanism was activated and whether the injury occurred before the protective mechanism was activated, during activation of the mechanism, or after activation of the mechanism, if applicable
- If the sharp had no engineered sharps injury protection, the injured employee's opinion as to whether and how such a mechanism could have prevented the injury
- The employee's opinion about whether any other engineering, administrative, or work practice control could have prevented the injury

After an incident has been reported, your employer will need to identify and document the source individual and obtain consent and make arrangements to have the source individual tested as soon as possible to determine HIV, HCV, and HBV infection.

FYI

State Laws

State laws may vary. Please check with your instructor regarding testing and test result confidentiality laws in your state.

It may not always be feasible to identify the source individual. Examples of when you may be unable to identify the source individual include needlesticks caused by unmarked syringes left in laundry or those involving blood samples that are not properly labeled, as well as incidents occurring where state or local laws prohibit such identification.

As stated before, the source individual's blood (if available) may be tested for HBV, HCV, and/or HIV, and the results of the test will be made known to you. Testing of the source individual's blood may be performed after consent is obtained. It should be documented when legally required consent to test the blood is not obtained.

Your blood may be tested for HBV, HCV, and/or HIV only with your consent. You may refuse. Counseling and evaluation of reported illnesses are not dependent on you choosing to have baseline HBV, HCV,

and HIV serologic testing. The results of HIV testing must be made in person and cannot be given over the telephone or mail. OSHA encourages employees to consent to blood collection at the time of exposure.

You may choose to have your blood drawn and stored for 90 days. If you change your mind within the 90 days, testing will be done. The 90-day time frame allows you to have the opportunity to obtain knowledge about baseline serologic testing after exposure incidents and to participate in further discussion, education, or counseling. If you elect not to have the blood tested, the sample will be disposed of without testing after 90 days.

OSHA Tips

OSHA does not require redrawing of the source individual's blood specifically for HBV, HCV, and HIV testing without the consent of the source individual.

▶ Specific Bloodborne Pathogens

Hepatitis Viruses

Hepatitis means "inflammation of the liver." Hepatitis has a variety of causes, including drugs, poisons and other toxins, and bloodborne pathogens. This section will focus on three causes of viral hepatitis that are important in the United States: HAV, HBV, and HCV.

HAV

Hepatitis A is a liver disease caused by the hepatitis A virus. Hepatitis A can affect anyone. In the United States, hepatitis A can occur in situations ranging from isolated cases of disease to widespread epidemics.

Good personal hygiene and proper sanitation can help prevent hepatitis A. Vaccines are also available for long-term prevention of HAV infection in persons 12 months of age and older.

CAUTION

Infection with one form of hepatitis does not prevent infection with another form of hepatitis. For example, a person with an HCV infection may still become infected with HBV.

OSHA Tips
Include important information related to the OSHA Standard.

resource preview

Site-Specific Work Pages
Allow students to track their bloodborne pathogens training and ensure that the training meets the OSHA Standard.

22

Site-Specific Work Page

Employee Training

In addition to HBV, HBC, and HIV, the instructor also reviewed the following bloodborne pathogens.

Pathogen: _____

Prevention and Control: _____

Clinical Features and History of the Disease: _____

Postexposure Prophylaxis and Follow-up: _____

Pathogen: _____

Prevention and Control: _____

Clinical Features and History of the Disease: _____

Postexposure Prophylaxis and Follow-up: _____

Pathogen: _____

Prevention and Control: _____

Clinical Features and History of the Disease: _____

Postexposure Prophylaxis and Follow-up: _____

The required medical records are maintained by: _____

at (location): _____

Medical records are kept for the duration of my employment plus 30 years: ☐ Yes   ☐ No

Medical care at my worksite is provided by: _____

Medical records are provided to you or to anyone having written consent from you within 15 days: ☐ True   ☐ False

The person responsible to evaluate if an exposure incident meets OSHA record keeping requirements is: _____

Hepatitis B vaccine is provided by _____ at (location)

The health professional's written opinion concerning hepatitis B immunization is limited to whether the employee requires the vaccine and whether the vaccine was administered: ☐ True   ☐ False

My question about Hepatitis B is: _____

My question about Hepatitis C is: _____

My question about HIV is: _____

My question about another bloodborne pathogen is: _____

Prep Kit
End-of-chapter resources that help reinforce important concepts and improve students' comprehension.
Vital Vocabulary: List of the key terms and definitions from the chapter.
Check Your Knowledge: Quiz students on the chapter's core concepts.

23

prep kit

▶ Vital Vocabulary

AIDS Acquired immunodeficiency syndrome; a disease that results from HIV.

antigen A substance that causes antibody formation.

hepatitis A A liver disease caused by the hepatitis A virus. Hepatitis A does not cause chronic disease.

hepatitis C A viral infection of the liver that is transmitted primarily by exposure to blood. Currently there is no vaccine effective against HCV.

immune Resistant to infectious disease.

immunization A process or procedure by which resistance to infectious disease is produced in a person.

jaundice A yellowing of the skin associated with hepatitis infection.

mucous membrane Any one of the four types of thin sheets of tissue that cover or line various parts of the body. An example would be the skin lining the nose and mouth.

percutaneous Performed through the skin as in draining fluid from an abscess using a needle.

source individual Any individual, living or dead, whose blood or other potentially infectious materials may be a source of occupational exposure to the employee. Examples include, but are not limited to, hospital and clinic patients; clients in institutions for the developmentally disabled; trauma victims; clients of drug and alcohol treatment facilities; residents of hospices and nursing homes; human remains; and individuals who donate or sell blood or blood components.

▶ Check Your Knowledge

1. For which virus is there an effective vaccine?
   A. HIV
   B. HCV
   C. HBV

2. If you do not respond to the first HBV immunization series you may be revaccinated with a second series.
   A. True
   B. False

3. List two symptoms of hepatitis.

4. Symptoms are not helpful in diagnosing HIV infection.
   A. True
   B. False

5. HIV is the virus that causes AIDS.
   A. True
   B. False

6. Antiviral medications and protease inhibitors are used in the treatment of HCV and HIV.
   A. True
   B. False

7. It is necessary to report as much detail as possible about an exposure incident.
   A. True
   B. False

8. Hepatitis B vaccine is offered at no cost to you.
   A. True
   B. False

9. Hepatitis C virus causes chronic liver disease in 70% of the people infected.
   A. True
   B. False

10. A liver transplant may be necessary to treat a chronic infection with hepatitis C.
    A. True
    B. False

11. It is possible to diagnose infection with HIV, HBV, and HCV with a blood test.
    A. True
    B. False

12. Infection with bloodborne pathogens occurs primarily through puncture injuries.
    A. True
    B. False

Jones and Bartlett would like to thank the following people for their contributions to this text.

Karen Carruthers, RN
Senior Technical Writer
Exactis.com
Denver, Colorado

Mark Jackson, MD
President, Mind Body Medicine of Maine, PA
Bangor, Maine

Sally McKinnon, MPA, BSN
Chief Clinical Operations Officer
Penobscot Community Health Care
Bangor, Maine

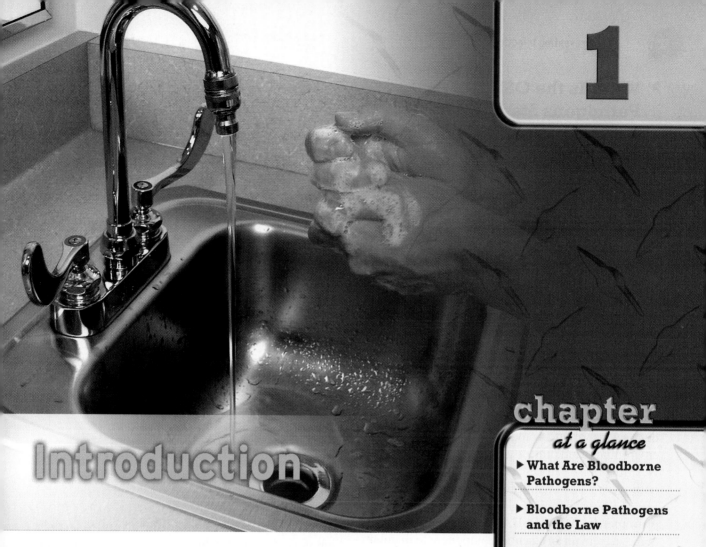

Introduction

▶ What Are Bloodborne Pathogens?

<u>Bloodborne pathogens</u> are disease-causing microorganisms (such as viruses, bacteria, or parasites) carried in human <u>blood</u>. Common bloodborne pathogens include hepatitis B, hepatitis C, and human immunodeficiency virus (HIV). These pathogens may be transmitted through unprotected contact with human blood or body fluids.

▶ Bloodborne Pathogens and the Law

Because certain jobs may involve contact with blood or other body fluid, the U.S. Department of Labor's Occupational Safety and Health Administration (OSHA) issued regulations to protect employees from bloodborne pathogens. These regulations are known as the OSHA Bloodborne Pathogens Standard, and they are designed to ensure employee safety through proper training and education, safety and prevention measures, and exposure control.

This text meets all current requirements of the OSHA Bloodborne Pathogens Standard.

▶ What Is the OSHA Bloodborne Pathogens Standard?

The OSHA Bloodborne Pathogens Standard (also referred to as 29 CFR 1910.1030) was issued in 1991 to protect employees from occupational exposure to bloodborne pathogens **Figure 1-1**. These regulations require employers to use a combination of engineering and work practice controls, personal protective clothing and equipment, medical surveillance, and additional safety precautions in the workplace. Any employees who are required to handle human blood or other potentially infectious materials (OPIMs) must receive training in bloodborne pathogens as well as onsite training to implement the requirements of specific work environments properly.

The standard has greatly improved employee safety through training and prevention measures. It has also influenced manufacturers to introduce new engineering controls (such as needleless systems) and produce a wide variety of products that create a safer work environment and provide greater personal protection. Despite these advances, however, bloodborne pathogens pose a significant occupational health risk for employees handling blood or OPIMs, and the requirements of the OSHA Bloodborne Pathogens Standard remain an essential component to maintaining a safe working environment. Appendix A gives the full text of the OSHA Bloodborne Pathogens Standard.

OSHA Bloodborne Pathogens Standard

OSHA Bloodborne Pathogens Regulations Section 1910.1030

Part 1910-[Amended]

Subpart Z-[Amended]

1. The general authority citation for subpart Z of 29 CFR part 1910 continues to read as follows and a new citation for 1910.1030 is added:

Authority: Secs. 6 and 8, Occupational Safety and Health Act, 29 U.S.C. 655, 657, Secretary of Labor's Orders Nos. 12-71 (36 CFR 8754), 8-76 (41 CFR 25059), or 9-83 (48 CFR 35736), as applicable; and 29 CFR part 1911.

* * *

Section 1910.1030 also issued under 29 U.S.C. 853.

* * *

2. Section 1910.1030 is added to read as follows:

1910.1030 Bloodborne Pathogens.

(a) Scope and Application

This section applies to all occupational exposure to blood or other potentially infectious materials as defined by paragraph (b) of this section.

(b) Definitions

For purposes of this section, the following shall apply:

Assistant Secretary means the Assistant Secretary of Labor for Occupational Safety and Health, or designated representative.

Blood means human blood, human blood components, and products made from human blood.

Bloodborne Pathogens means pathogenic microorganisms that are present in human blood and can cause disease in humans. These pathogens include, but are not limited to, Hepatitis B Virus [HBV] and Human Immunodeficiency Virus [HIV].

Clinical Laboratory means a workplace where diagnostic or other screening procedures are performed on blood or other potentially infectious materials.

Contaminated means the presence or the reasonably anticipated presence of blood or other potentially infectious materials on an item or surface.

Contaminated Laundry means laundry which has been soiled with blood or other potentially infectious materials or may contain sharps.

Contaminated Sharps means any contaminated object that can penetrate the skin including, but not limited to, needles, scalpels, broken glass, broken capillary tubes, and exposed ends of dental wires.

Decontamination means the use of physical or chemical means to remove, inactivate, or destroy bloodborne pathogens on a surface or item to the point where they are no longer capable of transmitting infectious particles and the surface or item is rendered safe for handling, use, or disposal.

Director means the Director of the National Institute for Occupational Safety and Health, U.S. Department of Health and Human Services, or designated representative.

Engineering Controls means controls (e.g., sharps disposal containers, self-sheathing needles) that isolate or remove the bloodborne pathogens hazard from the workplace.

Exposure Incident means a specific eye, mouth, other mucous membrane, non-intact skin, or parenteral contact with blood or other potentially infectious materials that results from the performance of an employee's duties.

Handwashing Facilities means a facility providing an adequate supply of running potable water, soap, and single use towels or hot air drying machines.

Licensed Health Care Professional is a person whose legally permitted scope of practice allows him or her to independently perform the activities required by paragraph (f) Hepatitis B vaccination and Post-Exposure Evaluation and Follow-Up.

HBV means Hepatitis B Virus.

HIV means Human Immunodeficiency Virus.

Occupational Exposure means reasonably anticipated skin, eye, mucous membrane, or parenteral contact with blood or other potentially infectious materials that may result from the performance of an employee's duties.

Other Potentially Infectious Materials means

(1) The following human body fluids: semen, vaginal secretions, cerebrospinal fluid, synovial fluid, pleural fluid, pericardial fluid, peritoneal fluid, amniotic fluid, saliva in dental procedures, any body fluid that is visibly contaminated with blood, and all body fluids in situations where it is difficult or impossible to differentiate between body fluids;

(2) Any unfixed tissue or organ (other than intact skin) from a human (living or dead); and

(3) HIV-containing cell or tissue cultures, organ cultures, and HIV- or HBV-containing culture medium or other solutions; and blood, organs, or other tissues from experimental animals infected with HIV or HBV.

Parenteral means piercing mucous membranes or the skin barrier through such events as needlesticks, human bites, cuts, and abrasions.

Figure 1-1

OSHA Bloodborne Pathogen Standard.

▶ Who Needs OSHA Bloodborne Pathogens Training?

The scope of the standard is not limited to employees with job classifications that may have occupational exposure to blood and OPIMs. For example, employees trained in first aid and identified by their employer as responsible for administering medical assistance on the job need to receive training in bloodborne pathogens.

The standard includes the potential for exposure, not just actual exposure. For example, emergency department intake personnel may not have an actual exposure to a bleeding patient, but the potential for exposure may exist.

OSHA Tips — **CALIFORNIA**

CalOSHA is the California Occupational Safety and Health Administration, which is responsible for ensuring the safety and health of California employees. Throughout the text, California participants may wish to refer to the boxes, which indicate CalOSHA standards that differ from federal OSHA requirements.

Employees

Any employee who has occupational exposure to blood or OPIMs is included within the scope of the standard. This includes part-time, temporary health care workers known as "per diem" employees and volunteers.

OSHA jurisdiction extends only to private business employees in the workplace. It does *not* extend to the following:

- Students if they are not considered an employee (students participating in internships are covered)

- State, county, or municipal employees
- Health care professionals who are sole practitioners or partners
- Those who are self-employed

Any employee who has potential for occupational exposure to blood or OPIMs is required to receive training **Figure 1-2** . The following job classifications may be associated with tasks that have occupational exposure to blood or OPIMs, but the standard is not limited to employees in these positions:

- Physicians, physician's assistants, nurses, nurse practitioners, and other health care employees in clinics and physicians' offices
- Employees of clinical and diagnostic laboratories
- Housekeepers in health care and other facilities
- Personnel in hospital laundries or commercial laundries that service health care or public-safety institutions
- Tissue bank personnel
- Employees in blood banks and plasma centers who collect, transport, and test blood
- Freestanding clinic employees (eg, hemodialysis clinics, urgent care clinics, health maintenance organization clinics, and family planning clinics)

- Employees in clinics in industrial, educational, and correctional facilities (eg, those who collect blood and clean and dress wounds)
- Employees designated to provide emergency first aid
- Dentists, dental hygienists, dental assistants, and dental laboratory technicians
- Staff of institutions for the developmentally disabled
- Hospice employees
- Home health care workers
- Staff of nursing homes and long-term care facilities
- Employees of funeral homes and mortuaries
- <u>Human immunodeficiency virus (HIV)</u> and <u>hepatitis B virus (HBV)</u> research laboratory and production facility workers
- Employees handling <u>regulated waste</u>; custodial workers required to clean up <u>contaminated sharps</u> or spills of blood or OPIMs
- Medical equipment service and repair personnel
- Emergency medical technicians, paramedics, and other emergency medical service providers
- Fire fighters, law enforcement personnel, and correctional officers
- Maintenance workers (eg, plumbers) in health care facilities and employees of substance abuse clinics

Employers and Employment Agencies

Employment agencies are not required to provide training because the agency is not considered the employer. The company or institution that uses the workers (such as a hospital) therefore is responsible for providing training according to the standard.

Personnel Services and Multiemployer Worksite Guidelines

Personnel service firms employ medical care staff who are assigned to work at hospitals and other health care facilities that contract with the firm. Often the employees are paid by the personnel services firm, but day-to-day supervision of the work is provided by the medical facility. When the medical facility (host employer) exercises day-to-day supervision over the personnel services worker, the worker is the employee of the host employer *and* the personnel service. The

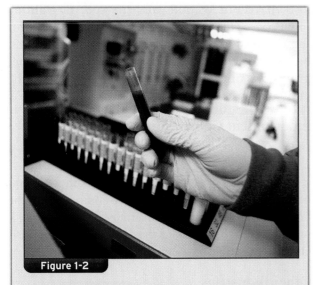

Figure 1-2

Any employee who has potential for occupational exposure to blood or OPIMs is required to receive training.

shared responsibilities of both employers are referred to as multiemployer worksite guidelines.

Under these circumstances, the personnel service firm can be held accountable for meeting the following provisions of the standard:

- Providing hepatitis B vaccinations
- Managing postexposure evaluation and follow-up
- Keeping records
- Providing generic training
- Exercising reasonable diligence to ensure that the host workplace facility is in compliance with the standard
- When violations of the standard at the host workplace are known, taking reasonable steps to have the host employer correct the violation

The host employer must comply with all provisions of the standard, such as providing appropriate engineering controls, an exposure control plan that is clearly explained and available to the worker, and personal protective equipment in the appropriate size and type. The host employer is obligated to take reasonable measures to ensure that the personnel service firm has complied with the provisions listed above.

Home Health Services

The employees of home health service companies may provide health services in private homes. Because the employer does not control the home work environment, the application of the bloodborne pathogens standard is restricted in the home health services industry.

The private home work environment is not free from bloodborne pathogen hazards, however. Employees should follow work practice guidelines and use personal protective equipment to prevent exposure.

OSHA has determined that the employer will not be held responsible for the following site-specific violations (such as violations occurring in a private home):

- Housekeeping requirements, such as the maintenance of a clean and sanitary worksite
- Handling and disposal of regulated waste
- Ensuring the use of personal protective equipment

- Ensuring that specific work practices are followed (such as handwashing with running water)
- Ensuring the use of engineering controls

The employer will be held responsible for all non–site-specific requirements of the standard, such as the following:

- The non–site-specific requirements of the exposure control plan
- Providing hepatitis B vaccinations
- Postexposure evaluation and follow-up
- Record keeping
- Providing generic training that is not workplace specific in detail and content
- Providing appropriate personal protective equipment to employees

Physicians and Health Care Professionals in an Independent Practice

Physicians may be employers or employees. In applying the provisions of the standard in situations involving physicians, the status of the physician is important. The responsibilities under the standard are similar to those of personnel services firms.

In general, professional corporations are the employers of their physician-members when they work at host employer sites and must comply with the hepatitis B vaccination, postexposure evaluation and follow-up, record keeping, and site-specific training provisions. The host employer is not responsible for these provisions for physicians with staff privileges, but the host employer must comply with all other provisions of the standard in accordance with the multiemployer worksite guidelines.

Independent Contractors

Independent contractors provide a service, such as a radiology service, to host employers. These contractors provide supervisory personnel and other personnel to carry out a service. Both the company and the host employer are responsible for complying with all provisions of the standard in accordance with multiemployer worksite guidelines.

Other Industries

The bloodborne pathogens standard does not apply to the construction, agricultural, marine terminal, and longshoring industries, although these industries are not free from the hazards of bloodborne pathogens.

Good Samaritan Assistance

Employees who do not fall within the scope of the standard may still experience a specific <u>exposure incident</u> at work that is unrelated to the performance of their job duties. An employee may choose to aid another person who is injured or ill, which is considered Good Samaritan assistance.

> ### FYI
>
> Good Samaritan acts are not covered under the standard.

> ### OSHA Tips
>
> OSHA strongly encourages employers to offer any employee who experiences an exposure incident at work confidential medical evaluation, including necessary postexposure prophylaxis and follow-up treatment.

▶ Why Do I Need This Manual?

This manual provides OSHA-specific bloodborne pathogens guidelines and is used with your worksite-specific training. You are encouraged to gather worksite-specific details on various work pages throughout the manual. Exercises at the end of each chapter help you check what you have learned and how it may be applied to your particular worksite requirements.

This manual will not make you an expert in bloodborne pathogens or the treatment of diseases caused by bloodborne pathogens. The manual does give you important and necessary information as required by the OSHA Bloodborne Pathogens Standard. Your instructor may expand on the information according to worksite-specific practices. The OSHA-required categories of information on page 6 must be included in all training.

▶ Meeting OSHA Standards

The goal of training is to educate employees regarding bloodborne pathogen issues and how to minimize or eliminate the exposure to bloodborne pathogens by using a combination of <u>universal precautions</u>, work practice controls, engineering controls, and personal protective equipment.

Employees being trained must have direct access to a qualified trainer. Educating employees solely by means of a film, video, or computer CD-ROM without the opportunity for a discussion period is not acceptable and constitutes a violation of the standard. The trainer must be familiar with the manner in which the elements in the training program relate to the workplace practices. This may also be accomplished by having two trainers: one to discuss generic bloodborne pathogen issues and one to discuss site-specific information **Figure 1-3** .

All employees at the time of initial assignment to tasks with occupational exposure to blood or OPIMs, before actually performing any of the tasks, must receive training on the hazards associated with blood and OPIMs and the protective measures to be taken to minimize the risk of occupational exposure.

Thereafter, training is provided at least annually and must be provided within 1 year of the original training. Whenever a change in an employee's responsibilities, procedures, or work situation is such that

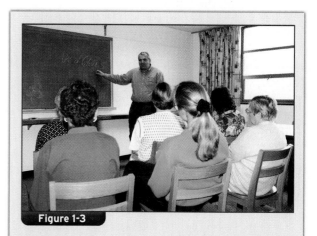

Figure 1-3

Annual training is necessary to ensure employee safety.

an employee's occupational exposure is affected, additional training or, as stated in the standard, "retraining" must take place. Retraining is not the same as annual training. Retraining must occur when new equipment is brought to the worksite that might affect the employee's possible exposure.

Annual training must cover the topics listed in the standard to the extent needed and must emphasize new information or procedures. In other words, if individuals are sitting through their fifth renewal class, the instructor may not need to cover the material to the depth that would be required in an initial training. Additionally, the course should be tailored to the group that the instructor is teaching.

The provisions for employee training are based on the employee's job responsibilities, with flexibility in training permitted to allow the program to be tailored to the employee's background and responsibilities or other site-specific needs. The categories of information presented in this manual must be included in any and all training.

OSHA requires that any training (including written material, oral presentations, films, videotapes, computer programs, or audiotapes) be presented in the employee's language and at the employee's education level. The trainer or an interpreter may convey the information.

It is necessary to record information about the dates of training sessions, a summary of the training content, and the names and job titles of the employees who attend the training.

OSHA Tips

Records that document employee training assist the employer and OSHA in determining whether the training program adequately addresses the risks involved in each job.

▶ OSHA-Required Categories of Information

A. An accessible copy of the Standard (Appendix A) and an explanation of its contents (this manual)
B. A general explanation of the epidemiology and symptoms of bloodborne disease (Chapter 2)
C. An explanation of the modes of transmission of bloodborne pathogens (Chapter 2)
D. An explanation of the employer's exposure control plan and the means by which the employee can obtain a copy of the written plan (supplied by your company directly or through the instructor) (Chapter 4)
E. An explanation of the appropriate methods for recognizing tasks and other activities that may involve exposure to blood and OPIMs (Chapter 3)
F. An explanation of the use and limitations of methods that will prevent or reduce exposure, including appropriate engineering controls, work practices, and personal protective equipment (Chapter 3)
G. An explanation of the requirements to evaluate, select, and use needleless systems and **sharps** with engineered **sharps injury** protections, which requires employee input, appropriate to circumstances of the workplace (Chapter 3)
H. Information on the types, proper use, location, removal, handling, **decontamination**, and disposal of personal protective equipment (Chapter 3)
I. An explanation of the basis for selection of personal protective equipment (Chapter 3)
J. Information on the hepatitis B **vaccine**, including information on its efficacy, safety, method of administration, the benefits of being vaccinated, and that the vaccine and vaccination will be offered free of charge to employees covered by the standard (Chapter 2)
K. Information on the appropriate actions to take and persons to contact in an emergency (exposure outside the normal scope of work) involving blood or OPIMs (Chapter 2)

L. An explanation of the procedure to follow if an exposure incident occurs, including the method of reporting the incident and the medical follow-up that will be made available (Chapter 2)

M. Information on the postexposure evaluation and follow-up that the employer is required to provide for the employee following an exposure incident (Chapter 2)

N. An explanation of the signs, labels, and/or color coding required (Chapter 3)

O. An opportunity for interactive questions and answers with the person conducting the training session (during and after training session)

▶ The Ryan White Act

The Centers for Disease Control and Prevention is in the process of preparing the final list of diseases required by the passage of the Public Law 101-381, the Ryan White Comprehensive AIDS Resources Emergency Act. The act creates a notification system for emergency response employees listed as police, fire, and EMS who are exposed to diseases such as *M tuberculosis*, hepatitis B or hepatitis C, and HIV.

▶ OSHA-Required Record Keeping

Record keeping needs to comply with 29 CFR 1904 using *Log of Work-Related Injuries and Illness* (Form 300) and *Injury and Illness Incident Report* (Form 301) and must record the following:

1. Any needlestick injury or cut from a sharp object that is contaminated with another person's blood or OPIMs

2. Any case requiring an employee to be medically removed under the requirements of an OSHA health standard

3. Tuberculosis infection as evidenced by a positive skin test or diagnosis by a physician or other licensed health care professional after exposure to a known case of active TB

This is in accordance with CPL2-0.131, effective January 1, 2002.

Additionally, there must be a <u>sharps injury log</u> maintained independently from the OSHA 300. This log must be confidential, and person-specific data should not be contained on the sharps injury log. At a minimum, the log must record the type and brand of the device involved, department or area of incident, and description of incident. The log should be reviewed on a regular basis, and action should be taken to correct any problems that are leading to needlestick or sharps injury.

FYI

Sharps Injury Logs
The employer must maintain records in a way that segregates sharps injuries from other types of work-related injuries.

Site-Specific Work Page

Employee Training

Date/Time of Training _____

Training Location _____

Your Name _____

This bloodborne pathogens training has been conducted by: _____

Attach a few comments about his or her qualifications. _____

_____

Name of your supervisor or other responsible person you would contact in the event of an exposure.

_____

BBP training materials are available at: _____

This is: ___ Initial training: ☐ Yes ☐ No ___ Retraining: ☐ Yes ☐ No ___ Annual training: ☐ Yes ☐ No

This training occurred during my routine work hours: ☐ Yes   ☐ No

This training occurred at no cost to me: ☐ Yes   ☐ No

A copy of the standard is included in my bloodborne pathogens manual: ☐ Yes   ☐ No

The training materials used by the instructor are easy for me to understand: ☐ Yes   ☐ No

The training materials used are in a language I understand: ☐ Yes   ☐ No

Terms are defined in Appendix A of my bloodborne pathogens manual: ☐ Yes   ☐ No

My company's exposure control plan is available at: _____

Training records are available for 3 years and are kept by: _____

I may request a copy of my training record from: _____

Request for a copy of my training record is to be provided within 15 days: ☐ Yes   ☐ No

Training records are not considered confidential: ☐ Yes   ☐ No

Questions about the standard were answered by the trainer: ☐ Yes   ☐ No

My question about the OSHA Bloodborne Pathogens Standard is: _____

▶ Vital Vocabulary

blood The term "human blood components" includes plasma, platelets, and serosanguinous fluids (eg, exudates from wounds). Also included are medications derived from blood, such as immune globulins, albumin, and factors 8 and 9.

bloodborne pathogens While HBV and HIV are specifically identified in the standard, the term includes any pathogenic microorganism that is present in human blood or OPIMs and can infect and cause disease in persons who are exposed to blood containing the pathogen.

contaminated sharps Any contaminated object that can penetrate the skin including, but not limited to, needles, scalpels, broken capillary tubes, and exposed ends of dental wires.

decontamination The use of physical or chemical means to remove, inactivate, or destroy bloodborne pathogens on a surface or item to the point where they are no longer capable of transmitting infectious particles and the surface or item is rendered safe for handling, use, or disposal.

engineering controls Physical controls (eg, sharps disposal containers, self-sheathing needles, safer medical devices such as sharps with engineered sharps injury protections and needleless systems) that isolate or remove the bloodborne pathogens hazard from the workplace. *Engineered sharps injury protection* means either: (1) A physical attribute built into a needle device used for withdrawing body fluids, accessing a vein or artery, or administering medications or other fluids, which effectively reduces the risk of an exposure incident by a mechanism such as barrier creation, blunting, encapsulation, withdrawal, or other effective mechanisms; or (2) A physical attribute built into any other type of needle device, or into a non-needle sharp, which effectively reduces the risk of an exposure incident.

exposure incident A specific eye, mouth, other mucous membrane, non-intact skin, or parenteral contact with blood or other potentially infectious materials that results from the performance of an employee's duties.

hepatitis B virus (HBV) One of the viruses that causes illness directly affecting the liver. It is a bloodborne pathogen.

human immunodeficiency virus (HIV) A virus that infects immune system blood cells in humans and renders them less effective in preventing disease.

medical surveillance A periodic comprehensive review of employees' health status as it relates to their potential exposures to hazardous agents.

needleless systems Devices that do not utilize needles for: (1) The withdrawal of body fluids after initial venous or arterial access is established; (2) The administration of medication or fluids; and (3) Any other procedure involving the potential for an exposure incident.

occupational exposure Reasonably anticipated skin, eye, mucous membrane, or parenteral contact with blood or other potentially infectious materials that may result from the performance of an employee's duties. "Reasonably anticipated contact" includes, among others, contact with blood or OPIM (including regulated waste) as well as incidents of needlesticks.

other potentially infectious materials (OPIMs) Coverage under this definition also extends to blood and tissues of experimental animals that are infected with HIV or HBV.

personal protective equipment Specialized clothing or equipment worn or used by an employee for protection against a hazard. General work clothes (eg, uniforms, pants, shirts or blouses) not intended to function as protection against a hazard are not considered to be personal protective equipment.

regulated waste Liquid or semi-liquid blood or other potentially infectious materials; contaminated items that would release blood or other potentially infectious materials in a liquid or semi-liquid state if compressed; items that are caked with dried blood or other potentially infectious materials and are capable of releasing these materials during handling; contaminated sharps; and pathological and microbiological wastes containing blood or other potentially infectious materials.

prep kit

sharps Any objects used or encountered in the industries covered by subsection (a) that can be reasonably anticipated to penetrate the skin or any other part of the body, and to result in an exposure incident, including, but not limited to, needle devices, scalpels, lancets, broken glass, broken capillary tubes, exposed ends of dental wires and dental knives, drills, and burs.

sharps injury Any injury caused by a sharp, including, but not limited to, cuts, abrasions, or needlesticks.

sharps injury log A written or electronic record satisfying the requirements of subsection (c)(2).

universal precautions An approach to infection control. According to the concept of Universal Precautions, all human blood and certain human body fluids are treated as if known to be infectious for HIV, HBV, HCV, and other bloodborne pathogens.

vaccine A suspension of inactive or killed microorganisms administered orally or injected into a human to induce active immunity to infectious disease.

work practice controls Controls that reduce the likelihood of exposure by altering the manner in which a task is performed (eg, prohibiting recapping of needles by a two-handed technique and use of patient-handling techniques).

▶ Check Your Knowledge

1. What kind of task would require training in bloodborne pathogens and OPIM safety? *blood draw*

2. An explanation of the symptoms caused by bloodborne pathogens is not a site-specific topic.
   A. True —
   B. False

3. Information about the locations of the eye wash stations is a site-specific topic.
   A. True
   B. False

4. Recommending and participating in the selection of engineering controls or personal protective equipment is an example of site-specific information.
   A. True
   B. False

5. There are no industries that are free from the hazards of bloodborne pathogens.
   A. True
   B. False

6. Name an industry not covered by the OSHA Bloodborne Pathogens Standard. *Agriculture*

7. If there is a change to my work practices that would change my exposure to bloodborne pathogens, I would receive retraining.
   A. True
   B. False

8. I must receive training every year.
   A. True
   B. False

9. OSHA requires the use of engineering controls.
   A. True
   B. False

10. The sharps injury log does not need to be kept confidential.
    A. True
    B. False

Answers: 1. Drawing blood, transporting blood, housekeeping in a health care facility; 2. A; 3. A; 4. A; 5. A; 6. Construction, agriculture, marine terminals, or longshore industries; 7. A; 8. A; 9. A; 10. B

Bloodborne Pathogens

▸ Overview

Occupational exposure to blood or other potentially infectious materials (OPIMs) means that you are at risk for infection from disease-causing organisms that may be transmitted through direct contact with blood or OPIMs. The hazard of exposure to infected blood or OPIMs is not restricted to the health care industry.

The likelihood of becoming infected after a single exposure to blood containing a disease-causing organism depends on many factors. The factors most commonly associated with transmission of disease include the presence of the organism in the source blood or OPIM, the type of injury or contact that you sustained (such as splash or puncture wound), the viral level present in the <u>source individual</u>, your current health (eg, if you have an illness that suppresses your immune system), and your immunization status (eg, if you are immunized against hepatitis B).

Many bloodborne pathogens exist. The likelihood of being exposed to a particular disease-causing organism varies and is affected by the following:

1. The geographic region where the work occurs (certain countries and/or areas have a much higher incidence of diseases caused by bloodborne pathogens). It is estimated that 16 to 18 million people in Central and

South America are infected with *Typanosoma cruzy,* a bloodborne pathogen parasite responsible for Chagas disease; however, unless you visit these countries or someone with the disease from these countries comes to the United States, the chance of contracting this disease is slim.

2. The type of work performed (eg, work in a research lab that investigates and cultures various viruses and bacteria may increase the risk).

It is not possible to include every possible bloodborne pathogen in this manual; therefore, the emphasis in this section is on the hepatitis B virus (HBV), hepatitis C virus (HCV), and HIV. The standard includes any pathogenic microorganism that may be present in human blood or OPIMs and that can infect and cause disease in persons who are exposed to blood containing the pathogen.

Your employer should determine whether to include information about other bloodborne pathogens in your training based on your geographic location and type of potential exposure. For example, if you work in facilities that are located near Mexico, you might reasonably expect to have occupational exposure to the blood of people from Mexico or Central America and need to learn more about Chagas disease.

▶ What Are Bloodborne Pathogens?

Bloodborne pathogens are disease-causing microorganisms (viruses, bacteria, and parasites) that may be present in human blood. They may be transmitted during exposure to blood or OPIMs.

▶ Mode of Transmission of Bloodborne Pathogens

Bloodborne pathogens are transmitted when blood or OPIMs come in contact with <u>mucous membranes</u> or nonintact skin. Nonintact skin includes, but is not limited to, cuts, abrasions, burns, rashes, acne, paper cuts, and hangnails. Bloodborne pathogens may also be transmitted by blood splashes or sprays, handling or touching contaminated items or surfaces, and injection under the skin by puncture wounds or cuts from contaminated sharps **Figure 2-1**.

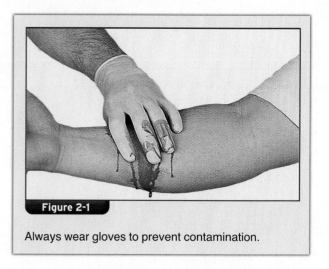

Figure 2-1

Always wear gloves to prevent contamination.

Most occupational transmission of HIV has occurred through puncture injuries from contaminated sharps; however, there have been documented transmissions through nonintact skin and mucous membranes. One worker became HIV positive after a splash of HIV-contaminated blood to the eyes. Contact with blood or OPIM should be avoided.

▶ OSHA Expectations Regarding Exposure

The objective of the standard is to minimize or eliminate the hazard posed by exposure to blood or OPIMs; however, occupational exposure to a bloodborne pathogen may occur.

If there is a risk of exposure or injury, it is important to know the following:

1. If there is a way to prevent infection as a result of exposure to the pathogen (such as <u>immunization</u>)
2. The symptoms caused by infection with the pathogen, as well as the natural course of the infection
3. Counseling specific to the exposure incident is available
4. The postexposure treatments and follow-up that may be provided

If you are exposed to bloodborne pathogens, a confidential medical evaluation is to be made *immediately* available to you, the injured employee. The word *immediately* is used in the standard to emphasize the importance of prompt medical evaluation and prophylaxis. An exact timeframe cannot be stated because the effectiveness of postexposure prophylactic measures varies depending on the infecting organism.

Medical evaluation must be confidential and protect your identity and test results.

FYI

Activities Associated With Sharps Injuries
Needlestick and other sharps injuries are primarily associated with the following activities: disposing needles; administering injections; drawing blood, including the use of glass capillary tubes; recapping needles; and handling trash and dirty linens.

If you go for a medical evaluation, the following information will be made available to the health professional:

1. A copy of the OSHA guidelines section 1910.1030. This is the OSHA standard that dictates the requirement for all aspects of bloodborne pathogens and infectious diseases. The OSHA standard provides the necessary procedures for the medical evaluation.
2. A description of how the incident occurred as it relates to your employment
3. The results of the source individual's testing (if available)
4. All medical records that are relevant for your proper treatment (if treatment is necessary), including a copy of your hepatitis B vaccination status with the dates of all the hepatitis B

FYI

Blood Testing Results
Employers do not have a specific right to know the actual results of the source individual's blood testing, but they must ensure that the information is provided to the evaluating health care professional.

---

vaccinations and any medical records relative to your ability to receive the vaccination

You and your employer should expect that current Centers for Disease Control and Prevention (CDC) guidelines will be used to guide postexposure prophylaxis and treatment.

It is the employer's responsibility to ensure that your medical records are kept confidential. Your records cannot be disclosed without your express written consent to any person within or outside the workplace, except as required by law. Your employer will have a copy of the health care provider's written opinion regarding the incident.

During consultation with the health care professional, decisions will be made about the need for hepatitis B vaccination, and laboratory tests and information will be provided about available postexposure prophylaxis and treatments.

The health care professional will discuss the laboratory test results with you. A plan will be created that identifies any necessary follow-up or treatments, including initiation of hepatitis B immunization, if indicated. Postexposure treatments and follow-up plans should be in accordance with the current CDC guidelines.

▶ Reporting Requirements

What Is an Occupational Exposure Incident?

An occupational exposure incident occurs if you are in a work situation and come in contact with blood or OPIM.

For OSHA 2000 record keeping purposes, an occupational bloodborne pathogens exposure incident (such as a needlestick, laceration, or splash) is classified as an *injury* because it is usually the result of an instantaneous event or exposure **Figure 2-2** .

After an occupational exposure to blood or OPIM has occurred, the employee's name and job classification are listed on the OSHA 2000 log. The job classification should be reviewed, and a determination should be made as to which employees, if any, in that classification should be covered under the standard.

OSHA Tips

As part of bloodborne pathogen training, OSHA requires that information on the appropriate actions to take and persons to contact in an emergency involving blood or OPIMs be provided.

Exposure Determination

The employer must identify and document the job classifications in which exposure occurs. The exposure determination must have been made without taking into consideration the use of personal protective clothing or equipment. The exposure control plan should identify the person responsible for the determination and assessment of an exposure incident.

Reporting an Incident

The goal of reporting an incident is to ensure that an employee receives timely access to medical services and to identify and adopt other methods or devices to prevent exposure incidents from recurring.

At sites where an exposure incident has occurred, it should be determined whether OSHA Standards were properly followed through interviews and reviews of incident reports or medical records.

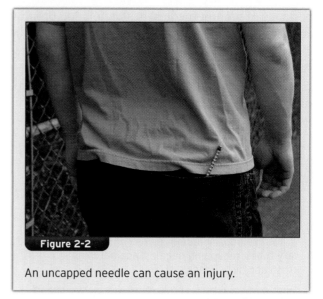

Figure 2-2

An uncapped needle can cause an injury.

OSHA Tips   CALIFORNIA

California OSHA requires a sharps injury log that records the date and time of each sharps injury resulting in an exposure incident, as well as the type and brand of device involved in the exposure incident.

FYI

Emergency Measures in the Event of an Exposure

- If you have an exposure incident to another person's blood or OPIM, immediately wash the exposed area with warm water and soap.
- If the exposed area was in your mouth, rinse your mouth with water or mouthwash (whichever is most readily available).
- If the exposure was in your eyes, flush with warm water (or normal saline if available). A quick rinse is probably not adequate; you want to irrigate the area completely with water.
- Your employer will have site-specific work practices to follow in event of an emergency.

The employee needs to report the incident to his or her supervisor. OSHA requires that the following information be reported:

- Date and time of the exposure incident
- Job classification of the exposed employee
- Worksite location where the exposure incident occurred
- Work practices being followed
- Engineering controls in use at the time including a description of the device in use (such as type and brand of sharp involved in the exposure incident)
- Protective equipment or clothing that was used at the time of the exposure incident
- Procedure being performed when the incident occurred
- Your training for the activity

The California OSHA also requires the following:

- Identifying the body part involved in the exposure incident
- The engineering controls in use at the time if the sharp had engineered sharps injury protection
- Whether the protective mechanism was activated and whether the injury occurred before the protective mechanism was activated, during activation of the mechanism, or after activation of the mechanism, if applicable
- If the sharp had no engineered sharps injury protection, the injured employee's opinion as to whether and how such a mechanism could have prevented the injury
- The employee's opinion about whether any other engineering, administrative, or work practice control could have prevented the injury

After an incident has been reported, your employer will need to identify and document the source individual and obtain consent and make arrangements to have the source individual tested as soon as possible to determine HIV, HCV, and HBV infection. It should be documented when legally required consent to test the blood is not obtained.

FYI

State Laws
State laws may vary. Please check with your instructor regarding testing and test result confidentiality laws in your state.

It may not always be feasible to identify the source individual. Examples of when you may be unable to identify the source individual include needlesticks caused by unmarked syringes left in laundry or those involving blood samples that are not properly labeled, as well as incidents occurring where state or local laws prohibit such identification.

Your blood may be tested for HBV, HCV, and/or HIV only with your consent. OSHA encourages employees to consent to blood collection at the time of exposure. The results of HIV testing must be made in person and cannot be given over the telephone or by mail. Even if you choose not to undergo testing, coun-seling and evaluation of reported illnesses are available to you.

You may choose to have your blood drawn but not tested and stored for 90 days. The 90-day time frame allows the employee to have the opportunity to obtain knowledge about baseline serologic testing after exposure incidents and to participate in further discussion, education, or counseling. If you elect not to have the blood tested, the sample will be disposed of after 90 days.

OSHA Tips

OSHA does not require redrawing of the source individual's blood specifically for HBV, HCV, and HIV testing without the consent of the source individual.

▶ Specific Bloodborne Pathogens

Hepatitis Viruses

Hepatitis means inflammation of the liver. Hepatitis has a variety of causes, including drugs, poisons and other toxins, and bloodborne pathogens. This section will focus on three causes of viral hepatitis: HAV, HBV, and HCV.

HAV

Hepatitis A is a viral disease caused by the hepatitis A virus. Hepatitis A can affect anyone. In the United States, hepatitis A can occur in isolated cases to widespread epidemics.

Good personal hygiene and proper sanitation can help prevent hepatitis A. Vaccines are also available for long-term prevention of HAV infection in persons 12 months of age and older.

CAUTION

Infection with one form of hepatitis does not prevent infection with another form of hepatitis. For example, a person with an HCV infection may still become infected with HBV.

Prevention and Control

Routine vaccination for HAV should occur in:

- All children 1 year (12 through 23 months) of age.
- Persons 1 year of age and older traveling to or working in countries with high or intermediate prevalence of HAV, such as those located in Central or South America, Mexico, Asia (except Japan), Africa, and eastern Europe. The CDC website provides additional information.
- Children and adolescents through 18 years of age who live in states or communities where routine vaccination has been implemented because of high disease incidence.
- Men who have sex with men.
- Persons who use street drugs.
- Persons with chronic liver disease.
- Persons who are treated with clotting factor concentrates.
- Persons who work with HAV-infected primates or who work with HAV in research laboratories.

The HAV vaccine may be recommended for children or adolescents in communities where outbreaks of hepatitis A are occurring. *Hepatitis A vaccine is not licensed for administration to children younger than 1 year.*

For children, the first dose should be given at 12 to 23 months of age. Children who are not vaccinated by 2 years of age can be vaccinated at later visits.

For travelers, the vaccine series should be started at least 1 month before traveling to provide the best protection. For others, the HAV vaccine series may be started whenever a person is at risk of infection.

Two doses of the vaccine are needed for lasting protection. These doses should be given at least 6 months apart. HAV vaccine may be given at the same time as other vaccines.

HBV

Hepatitis B can affect anyone. Each year in the United States, 140,000 to 320,000 people will become infected with the virus. Studies conducted by the CDC have shown a steady decline in the incidence of HBV infection. This decline is attributed to the widespread use of HBV vaccine and the implementation of other prevention methods, such as engineering and work practice controls, personal protective equipment, and universal precautions.

It is estimated that 1 to 1.25 million Americans are chronically infected with HBV.

Prevention and Control

The HBV vaccine has been available since 1982. The vaccine does not contain any live components. The vaccine is given in a series of three shots **Figure 2-3**.

Immunization

All people who have routine occupational exposure to blood or OPIM have the right to receive the immunization series against HBV at no personal expense. The standard includes temporary and part-time workers and volunteers.

There are several reasons why you may choose not to receive the HBV vaccine. Among the most common reasons are as follows:

1. Documentation exists that you have previously received the series.
2. Antibody testing reveals that you are immune.
3. Medical evaluation shows that vaccination is contraindicated.
4. You are allergic to any component of the vaccine.

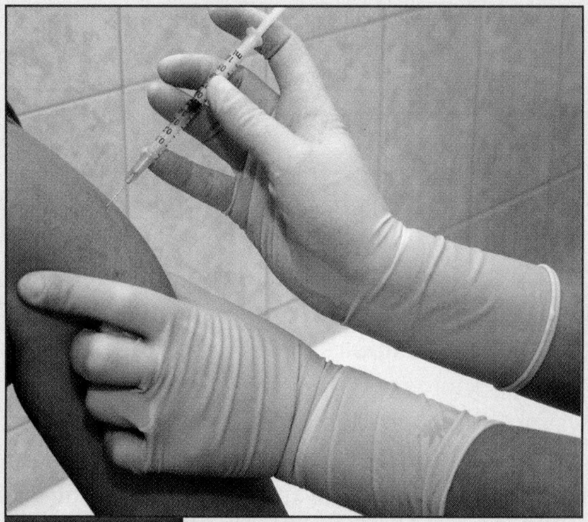

Figure 2-3

Immunization against HBV is possible.

Exception for HBV Vaccination

Designated first aid providers who have occupational exposure are not required to be offered HBV vaccine if the following conditions exist:

1. The primary job assignment of the designated first aid provider is not the rendering of first aid.
2. Any first aid rendered by the first aid provider is rendered only as a collateral duty responding solely to injuries resulting from workplace incidents and generally at the location where the incident occurred.
3. This provision does not apply to designated first aid providers who render assistance on a regular basis, for example, at a first aid station, clinic, dispensary, or other location where injured employees routinely go for such assistance, and emergency or public safety personnel who are expected to render first aid in the course of their work.

Prescreening antibody testing is not required, and your employer may not make prescreening a requirement for receiving the vaccine. If an employer wishes prescreening, it must be made available to you at no cost. If you choose to have prescreening, the testing must be done at an accredited laboratory.

The standard requires that your employer offer the vaccine at a convenient time and place to you, during normal work hours. If travel is required away from the worksite, your employer is responsible for that cost. The standard includes temporary and part-time workers.

Your employer cannot require you to pay for testing and then reimburse you if you remain employed for a specific time. Nor are you required to reimburse your employer for the cost of the vaccine if you leave your job.

FYI

HBV Vaccine

- Immunization with HBV vaccine should be made available within 10 working days of initial assignment to the job.
- Your employer cannot require you to use your health insurance or your family insurance to pay for the cost of the vaccine.
- To learn more about CDC recommendations visit http://www.cdc.gov/ncidod/dhqp/bp.html.

FYI

First Aid Providers

The employer's exposure control plan must specifically address the provisions of the standard as they apply to first aid providers.

The exposure control plan must include the following:

- Provision for a reporting procedure that ensures that all first aid incidents involving the presence of blood or OPIM will be reported to the employer before the end of the work shift during which the incident occurred.
- The report must include the names of all first aid providers who rendered assistance, regardless of whether personal protective equipment was used and must describe the first aid incident, including time and date. The description must include a determination of whether or not, in addition to the presence of blood or other potentially infectious materials, an "exposure incident," as defined by the standard, occurred. This determination is necessary in order to ensure that the proper postexposure evaluation, prophylaxis, and follow-up procedures required by the standard are made available immediately, whenever there has been an "exposure incident" as defined by the standard.
- A report that lists all such first aid incidents must be readily available, upon request, to all employees and to the assistant secretary.
- Provision for the bloodborne pathogens training program for designated first aid providers to include the specifics of this reporting procedure.
- Provision for the full hepatitis B vaccination series to be made available as soon as possible, but in no event later than 24 hours, to all unvaccinated first aid providers who have rendered assistance in any situation involving the presence of blood or OPIM, regardless of whether or not a specific "exposure incident," as defined by the standard, has occurred.

OSHA's intent is to have your employer eliminate obstacles to your acceptance of the vaccine; however, the term "made available" emphasizes that you may refuse the series by signing the HBV vaccine declination form (Appendix B). If you change your mind while still covered under the standard at a later date, you may still receive the vaccine at no cost.

If your job requires you to have ongoing contact with patients or blood and you are at ongoing risk for injuries with sharp instruments or needlesticks, the CDC recommends that you be tested for <u>antibody</u> to HBV surface <u>antigen</u> (HBsAg) 1 to 2 months after the completion of the three-dose vaccination series. If you do not respond to the primary vaccination series, you must be re-vaccinated with a second three-dose vaccine series and re-tested for HBsAg. Nonresponders must be medically evaluated.

Contraindications

You should not receive the vaccine if you are sensitive to yeast or any other component of the vaccine. Consultation with a physician is required for persons with heart disease, fever, or other illness. If you are pregnant or breastfeeding an infant, you should consult your physician before receiving the vaccine.

Side Effects of the Vaccine

The side effects of the vaccine are minimal and may include localized swelling, pain, bruising, or redness at the injection site. The most common systemic reactions include flu-like symptoms such as fatigue, weakness, headache, fever, or malaise.

About the Vaccines

Recombivax HB (Merck) or Engerix-B (GlaxoSmith-Kline Biologicals) are the vaccines used to prevent infection with the HBV. The vaccine against hepatitis B, prepared from recombinant yeast cultures, is free of association with human blood or blood products. In 1999, manufacturers began producing vaccines that are free of the preservative thimerosal. Thimerosal consists of approximately 50% mercury by weight and has raised toxicity concerns.

The vaccine is given in three doses over a 6-month period. The first is given at an agreed-on date and within 10 working days of the initial assignment; the second is given 1 month later, and the third dose is given 5 months after the second dose. The vaccine is administered by needle into a large muscle such as the deltoid in the upper arm; however, for persons at risk of hemorrhage after intramuscular injection, the vaccine may be administered subcutaneously.

In persons receiving the vaccine, 87% will develop immunity after the second dose of the vaccine, and 96% will develop immunity after the third dose.

Clinical Features and History of Hepatitis B

The symptoms of HBV infection typically last 4 to 6 weeks and include the following:

- <u>Jaundice</u> (your eyes or skin may turn yellow)
- Fatigue
- Abdominal pain
- Loss of appetite
- Intermittent nausea
- Vomiting

It is expected that 70,000 to 160,000 people will develop symptomatic infections with HBV, and 8,400 to 19,000 of these people will require hospitalization. Each year, as many as 320 persons will die of the acute infection with HBV.

The incubation period for HBV (the time from exposure to developing the disease) averages 12 weeks, with a range of 4 weeks to 6 months. In the majority (90% to 94%) of the cases, infection with HBV resolves without further complication; however, about 8,000 to 32,000 (6% to 10%) of all the annual infections will progress, and the individuals will suffer chronic infection with HBV. Over time, chronic infection causes significant injury to the liver; 5,000 to 6,000 deaths occur each year from chronic HBV liver disease.

Postexposure Prophylaxis and Follow-up for HBV

There is no cure for infection with HBV. HBV vaccination is the best protection.

All decisions about postexposure prophylaxis are made in consultation with your health care professional.

Postexposure treatment for HBV infection should begin within 24 hours and no later than 7 days.

The postexposure treatments available include HBV immunization and the use of immune globulin, which has been shown to be effective for passive immunization against HBV if given within hours after the exposure incident.

The decision to provide postexposure prophylaxis takes into account whether the source of the blood is available, the HBsAg status of the source blood, and the HBV vaccination and vaccine-response status of the exposed employee.

For any occupational exposure to blood or OPIM of a person not previously vaccinated, HBV vaccination is recommended.

The CDC reports that for an unvaccinated person, the risk from a single needlestick or cut exposure to HBV-infected blood ranges from 6% to 30% and depends on the hepatitis B e antigen (HBeAg) status of the source blood.

Chronic HBV infection treatment options include antiviral medications and/or liver transplantation.

HCV

Hepatitis C is the most common chronic bloodborne infection in the United States. HCV is transmitted primarily through large or repeated direct **percutaneous** exposures to blood (meaning passed through the skin).

The incidence of HCV infection has declined. Transfusion-associated cases occurred before blood donor screening and are now rare. Injectable drug abuse has accounted for a substantial proportion of HCV infections and currently accounts for 60% of HCV transmission in the United States.

It is estimated that 3.9 million Americans (1.8%) have been infected with HCV, of whom 2.7 million are chronically infected; 36,000 new infections occur in the United States each year.

Prevention and Control

There is no vaccination for HCV.

Prevention recommendations are directed toward the use of engineering and work practice controls, personal protective equipment, and universal precautions.

Clinical Features and History of Hepatitis C

Most patients (70% to 75%) with acute **hepatitis C** are asymptomatic. Symptoms may include the following:

> ## FYI
>
> ### Hepatitis C Virus
> - HCV has specifically been included wherever HIV and HBV are mentioned in the regulation.
> - The CDC reports that the prevalence of HCV infection among health care workers is no greater than the general population, averaging 1% to 2%, and is 10 times lower than the prevalence of HBV infection among health care workers.
> - Needlestick injury is the only occupational risk factor that has been associated with HCV infection.
> - Referral to a specialist in liver disease may be necessary to manage an infection with HCV properly.
> - In follow-up studies of health care workers who sustained percutaneous exposures to blood from anti-HCV-positive patients, the incidence of anti-HCV conversion averaged 3.5%.

- Jaundice (eyes or skin may turn yellow)
- Fatigue
- Abdominal pain
- Loss of appetite
- Intermittent nausea
- Vomiting

The incubation period (the time from exposure to developing the disease) averages 7 weeks (range, 3 to 20 weeks). Chronic infection is common, affecting more than 85% of people infected. Chronic liver disease may occur in 70% of those infected with HCV. It is estimated that 8,000 to 10,000 deaths occur each year as a result of HCV-associated liver disease. HCV is the major cause of liver disease requiring liver transplantation.

Postexposure Prophylaxis and Follow-up

There is no cure for infection with HCV.

All decisions about postexposure laboratory testing and prophylaxis are made in consultation with your health care professional. The test for HCV and liver function tests should occur as soon as possible after exposure and should be repeated at 4 to 6 months after the exposure.

Currently, there is no recommendation for post-exposure prophylaxis of HCV. Immune globulin is not effective in providing passive immunization against the disease.

When HCV infection is identified early, referral for medical management is necessary. Limited data indicate that antiviral therapy might be beneficial when started early in the course of the HCV infection; however, no guidelines currently exist for the use of antiviral medications in the acute phase of the infection.

The CDC reports that the risk for infection after a needlestick or cut exposure to HCV-infected blood is about 1.8%.

Chronic HCV infection treatment options include antiviral medications and liver transplantation.

HIV

Human immunodeficiency virus (HIV) is the virus that causes AIDS. Two types of HIV have been identified (HIV-1 and HIV-2). HIV infection causes suppression of the immune system and can lead to opportunistic infections and unusual types of cancer.

The differences between HIV-1 and HIV-2 should be noted. HIV-2 AIDS develops more slowly and may be milder. There are few reported cases of HIV-2 in the United States. HIV-2 is predominately found in Africa. Hereafter, all references to HIV mean HIV-1.

The CDC reports that in 2003 there were an estimated 1,039,000 people in the United States with HIV/AIDS. Approximately 25% of infected persons are undiagnosed and unaware of their infection.

The annual rate of infection with HIV is 16.5 cases per 100,000 population **Figure 2-4** .

Prevention and Control

There is no vaccination for HIV.

Prevention recommendations are directed toward the use of engineering and work practice controls, personal protective equipment, and universal precautions.

Clinical Features and History of HIV

The only way to determine for sure whether you are infected is to be tested. The incubation period with HIV from the time of HIV infection to the develop-

> ### FYI
> **Risk of HIV Infection From Percutaneous Exposure**
> The average risk for HIV infection from all types of reported percutaneous exposure to HIV infected blood is 0.3%.
> The risk is increased in exposures involving:
> - Deep injury to health care worker
> - Visible blood on the device causing the injury
> - A device previously placed in the source patient's vein or artery
> - A source patient who died as a result of AIDS within 60 days after exposure

> ### FYI
> **Antiviral Drugs**
> - Advances in the field of antiviral therapy and the use of protease inhibitors might change the recommendations for treatment and follow-up for HCV and HIV infection; therefore, it is important to work closely with your health care professional and use current CDC guidelines.
> - All antiviral drugs have been associated with significant side effects. Protease inhibitors may interact with other medications and cause serious side effects.

ment of AIDS may take 8 to 10 years. This time varies greatly from person to person.

You cannot rely on symptoms to know whether you are infected with HIV. Many people who are infected with HIV experience no symptoms for many years. The symptoms of AIDS are similar to the symptoms of many other infections and might include night sweats, weight loss, fever, fatigue, gland pain or swelling, and muscle or joint pain.

Postexposure Prophylaxis and Follow-up for HIV

There is no cure for infection with HIV.

All decisions about postexposure laboratory testing and prophylaxis are made in consultation with

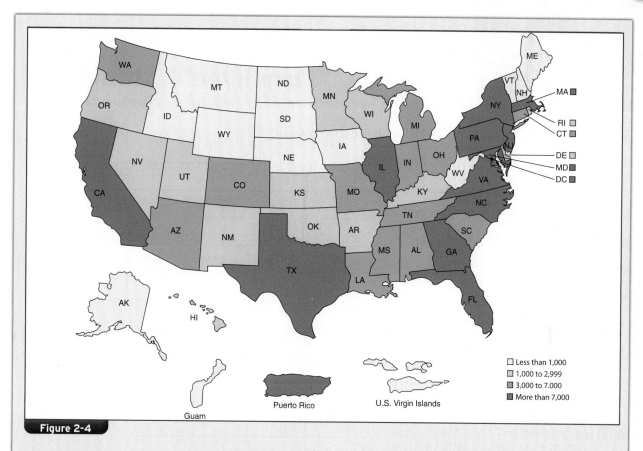

Figure 2-4

Estimated number of persons living with AIDS.

Source: The Kaiser Family Foundation, statehealthfacts.org. Data Source: HIV/AIDS Surveillance Report: Cases of HIV Infection and AIDS in the United States, 2005, Volume 16, National Center for HIV, STD and TB Prevention, Centers for Disease Control and Prevention, Department of Health and Human Services, 2006.

your health care professional. Testing for the HIV antibody should be done as soon as possible after exposure and, thereafter, periodically for at least 6 months. Antibodies usually become detectable within 3 months of infection.

Decisions regarding treatment need to be made after discussion with an infectious diseases specialist. Postexposure treatment is **not** recommended for all occupational exposures; 99.7% of the exposures do not lead to HIV infection. If treatment with antiviral medications plus a protease inhibitor is recommended, treatment should begin within hours of the exposure.

The CDC reports that the risk of infection after a needlestick or cut exposure to HIV-infected blood is about 0.3%.

Site-Specific Work Page

Employee Training

In addition to HBV, HBC, and HIV, the instructor also reviewed the following bloodborne pathogens.

Pathogen: _____

Prevention and Control: _____

Clinical Features and History of the Disease: _____

Postexposure Prophylaxis and Follow-up: _____

Pathogen: _____

Prevention and Control: _____

Clinical Features and History of the Disease: _____

Postexposure Prophylaxis and Follow-up: _____

Pathogen: _____

Prevention and Control: _____

Clinical Features and History of the Disease: _____

Postexposure Prophylaxis and Follow-up: _____

The required medical records are maintained by:_____

at (location): _____

Medical records are kept for the duration of my employment plus 30 years: ☐ Yes   ☐ No

Medical care at my worksite is provided by: _____

Medical records are provided to you or to anyone having written consent from you within 15 days: ☐ True   ☐ False

The person responsible to evaluate if an exposure incident meets OSHA record keeping requirements is:

_____

Hepatitis B vaccine is provided by _____ at (location) _____

The health professional's written opinion concerning hepatitis B immunization is limited to whether the employee requires the vaccine and whether the vaccine was administered: ☐ True   ☐ False

My question about Hepatitis B is: _____

My question about Hepatitis C is: _____

My question about HIV is: _____

My question about another bloodborne pathogen is: _____

▶ Vital Vocabulary

AIDS Acquired immunodeficiency syndrome; a disease that results from HIV.

antibody A specialized immune protein that binds to an antigen to make it more visible to the immune system.

antigen A substance that causes antibody formation.

hepatitis A A viral infection of the liver caused by the hepatitis A virus. Hepatitis A does not cause chronic disease.

hepatitis B A viral infection of the liver caused by the hepatitis B virus.

hepatitis C A viral infection of the liver that is transmitted primarily by exposure to blood. Currently there is no vaccine effective against HCV.

immune Resistant to infectious disease.

immunization A process or procedure by which resistance to infectious disease is produced in a person.

jaundice A yellowing of the skin associated with hepatitis infection.

mucous membrane Tissue lining body cavities such as the nose and mouth. It secretes mucus. Mucous membranes, unlike unbroken skin, can transmit some viruses such as hepatitis and HIV.

opportunistic infections Illnesses caused by various organisms, many of which often do not cause disease in persons with healthy immune systems.

percutaneous Occurring through the skin, such as drawing blood with a needle.

source individual Any individual, living or dead, whose blood or other potentially infectious materials may be a source of occupational exposure to the employee. Examples include, but are not limited to, hospital and clinic patients; clients in institutions for the developmentally disabled; trauma victims; clients of drug and alcohol treatment facilities; residents of hospices and nursing homes; human remains; and individuals who donate or sell blood or blood components.

▶ Check Your Knowledge

1. For which virus is there an effective vaccine?
   A. HIV
   B. HCV
   C. HBV —

2. If you do not respond to the first HBV immunization series you may be revaccinated with a second series.
   A. True _
   B. False

3. List two symptoms of hepatitis. *jaundice vomiting*

4. Symptoms are not specific in the diagnosis of HIV infection.
   A. True —
   B. False

5. HIV is the virus that causes AIDS.
   A. True —
   B. False

6. Post-exposure treatment of HIV and HCV is controversial and should be discussed with a physician immediately after exposure.
   A. True —
   B. False

7. It is necessary to report as much detail as possible about an exposure incident.
   A. True —
   B. False

8. Hepatitis B vaccine is offered at no cost to you.
   A. True —
   B. False

9. Hepatitis C virus causes chronic liver disease in 70% of the people infected.
   A. True —
   B. False

10. A liver transplant may be necessary to treat a chronic infection with hepatitis C.
    A. True —
    B. False

prep kit

11. It is possible to diagnose infection with HIV, HBV, and HCV with a blood test.

    A. True

    B. False

12. Infection with bloodborne pathogens occurs primarily through puncture injuries.

    A. True

    B. False

13. It is necessary to learn about other bloodborne pathogens.

    A. True

    B. False

14. Which virus poses the greatest risk for infection after a puncture injury?

    A. Hepatitis B or C

    B. HIV

15. More than one blood test is needed to determine whether there has been infection with HIV.

    A. True

    B. False

Answers: **1.** C; **2.** A; **3.** Jaundice, fever; **4.** A; **5.** A; **6.** A; **7.** A; **8.** A; **9.** A; **10.** A; **11.** A; **12.** A; **13.** B; **14.** B; **15.** A

Prevention

▶ Overview

The Occupational Safety and Health Administration (OSHA) defined four principal strategies to prevent or reduce exposure to bloodborne pathogens. These strategies are used in combination to offer you maximum protection. It is OSHA's view that preventing exposures requires a comprehensive program, including engineering controls (such as needleless devices, shielded needle devices, and plastic capillary tubes) and proper work practices (such as no-hands procedures in handling contaminated sharps). If engineering and work practice controls do not eliminate exposure, the use of personal protective equipment (PPE) (such as eye protection) and universal precautions is required.

Your employer's exposure control plan describes the engineering controls in use at your worksite. Significant improvements in technology are most evident in the growing market of safer medical devices that minimize, control, or prevent exposure incidents. Employee participation in the selection of new devices is required by OSHA. OSHA does not advocate the use of one particular device over another. An annual review of your employer's exposure control plan should include identification of new safety devices. Adoption of engineering controls requires changes to your employer's plan and retraining in the proper use of the control.

According to California OSHA, the use of needleless systems, needle devices with engineered sharps injury protection, and nonneedle sharps with engineered sharps injury protection is required except under four conditions:

1. Lack of market availability
2. Information that the device will jeopardize patient care
3. Information indicating that the device is not more effective in reducing sharps injuries than the device currently used by the employer
4. A lack of sufficient information to determine whether a new device on the market will effectively reduce the chances of a sharps injury

When the potential for exposure exists in spite of engineering and work practice controls, employers must provide PPE. *PPE* is used to protect you from contamination of skin or mucous membranes and puncture wounds. *Universal precautions* is a strategy to structure your approach to working with all human blood and certain body fluids. All of these strategies combined promote worker safety and provide a safer working environment.

▶ Engineering Controls

Engineering controls refers to any effort to design safety into the tools and workspace organization. Examples include handwashing facilities, eye stations, sharps containers, biohazard labels, self-sheathing needles on syringes, and needleless IV systems. Engineering controls include any object that comes between you and the potential infectious material.

Your employer is responsible for the full cost of instituting engineering and work practice controls. Your employer is also responsible for regularly examining and repairing and/or replacing engineering controls as often as necessary to ensure that each control

FYI

Engineering Controls
For situations in which engineering controls will reduce employee exposure by removing, eliminating, or isolating the hazard, they must be used.

OSHA Tips

Work practice controls must be evaluated and updated on a regular schedule to ensure their effectiveness. Your organization violates the standard if it fails to engage in effective monitoring.

is maintained and that it provides the protection intended. Regularly scheduled inspections are required to confirm, for instance, that engineering controls such as safer devices continue to function effectively, that protective shields have not been removed or broken, and that physical, mechanical, or replacement-dependent controls are functioning as intended. Your employer may assign this task to you.

Labeling Regulated Waste

What Is Regulated Waste?

The term *regulated waste* refers to the following categories of waste that require special handling, at a minimum:

- Liquid or semiliquid blood or other potentially infectious materials (OPIMs)
- Items contaminated with blood or OPIMs and that would release these substances in a liquid or semiliquid state if compressed
- Items that are caked with dried blood or OPIMs and are capable of releasing these materials during handling
- Contaminated sharps
- Pathological and microbiological wastes containing blood or OPIMs

When Is Labeling Regulated Waste Necessary?

Labels must be provided on containers of regulated waste, on refrigerators and freezers that are used to store blood or OPIMs, and on containers used to store, dispose of, transport, or ship blood or OPIMs.

Equipment that is being sent to another facility for servicing or decontamination must have a label attached stating which portions of the equipment remain contaminated to warn other employees of the hazard and encourage them to use proper precautions.

Labeling Regulated Waste

Regulated waste containers must be labeled with the biohazard label or color coded to warn individuals who may have contact with the containers of the potential hazard posed by their contents.

Even if your facility considers *all* of its waste to be regulated waste, the waste containers must still bear the required label or color coding in order to protect new employees and individuals and employees from outside facilities.

Regulated waste that has been decontaminated need not be labeled or color coded; however, your employer must have controls in place to determine whether the decontamination process is successful.

Blood and blood products that bear an identifying label as specified by the Food and Drug Administration and that have been screened for hepatitis B virus (HBV), hepatitis C virus (HCV), and HIV antibodies and released for transfusion or other clinical uses are exempted from the labeling requirements.

When blood is being drawn or laboratory procedures are being performed on blood samples, the individual containers housing the blood or OPIMs do not have to be labeled, provided the larger container into which they are placed for storage, transport, shipment, or disposal (such as a test tube rack) is labeled.

OSHA Tips

When there is an overlap between the OSHA-mandated label and the Department of Transportation (DOT)-required label, the DOT label will be considered acceptable on the outside of the transport container, provided that the OSHA-mandated label appears on any internal containers that may be present.

Biohazard Labels

Biohazard labels may be attached to bags containing potentially infectious materials. These labels must be fluorescent orange or orange-red with letters or symbols in a contrasting color. These are attached to any container that is used to store or transport potentially infectious materials Figure 3-1.

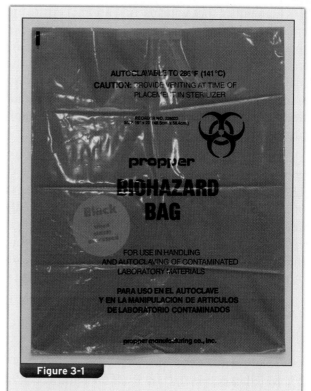

Figure 3-1

Biohazard labels may be attached to bags containing potentially infectious materials. The label must be fluorescent orange or orange-red in color and clearly visible.

The Needlestick Safety Prevention Act

The Needlestick Safety Prevention Act became effective April 2001 and requires employers to
- Implement new developments in control technology
- Solicit nonmanagerial employees with direct patient care who are exposed to these potential hazards for input in the identification, evaluation, and selection of engineering and work practice controls
- Maintain a log of percutaneous injuries from contaminated sharps

Specific procedures for obtaining employee input might include informal problem-solving groups, participation of employees in safety audits, workplace inspection, evaluation of devices, pilot testing devices, and membership on a committee that consistently meets to review and audit reports of these activities.

Remember that your participation is critical in creating a safe work environment. Participation in these activities ensures safer medical devices and the training to properly use these devices, as well as the identification of compatibility problems. In many instances, employee contribution has led to important decisions that result in the most appropriate engineered sharps being selected.

SESIP and Needleless Systems

The term SESIP or *Sharps with Engineered Sharps Injury Protections* means a needleless sharp or needle device used for withdrawing body fluids, accessing a vein or artery, or administering medications or other fluids with built-in safety features that effectively reduce the risk of an exposure incident **Figure 3-2**.

SESIP devices are available as
- Syringes with retractable needles
- Blunt-tipped blood-drawing needles
- Resheathing disposable scalpels
- Retracting finger prick lancets

Needleless systems are used for withdrawal of body fluids or administration of medications or fluids after the initial venous or arterial access is established or whenever a needleless system is available **Figure 3-3**.

FYI

Needles
Needles that will not become contaminated by blood during use (such as those used only to draw medication from vials) are not required to have engineering controls under the standard.

CAUTION

The standard prohibits the removal of contaminated needles from medical devices. When performing a blood-drawing procedure, it is necessary to dispose of the blood tube holder with a safety needle attached after each patient's blood is drawn.

Evaluating Safety Systems

Your employer must evaluate existing engineering and work practice controls and assess the feasibility of implementing new safety technology yearly. There are many new products introduced each year. Not all products may be correct for your work environment; however, these products should be evaluated with input from nonmanagerial employees who have patient care responsibilities. There are many new types of needleless systems. Examples of the new types of injection equipment, IV equipment, and laboratory equipment include the following:
- Needle guard—sliding sheath/sleeve
- Needle guard—hinged recap
- Needleless jet injection
- Retractable needles
- Needleless IV access—blunted cannulas
- Recessed protected needle
- Plastic blood collection tubes
- Self-blunting needle
- Lancets—laser and retracting
- Retracting scalpels
- Quick-release scalpel blade handles
- Blunted suture needle

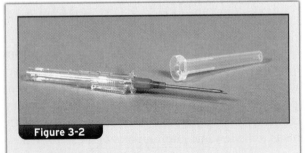

Figure 3-2

IV needle with auto sharp injury prevention.

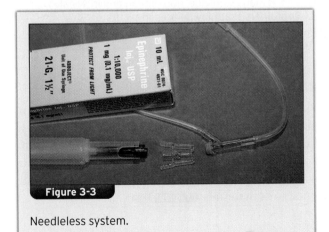

Figure 3-3

Needleless system.

The specific process for evaluating safety technology is not prescribed by the standard; however, experience has shown that a productive review process might include the following:

- Form a multidisciplinary team that follows a timetable for completing timely evaluations.
- Identify priority areas, and give the highest priority assessment to any <u>work area</u> or practice in which percutaneous injuries have occurred. Emphasize safety devices with features that will have the greatest impact on preventing occupational injury.
- Conduct the evaluation with participants who will actually use the selected device.
- Train the workers in the proper use of the device.
- Establish clear criteria and measures for evaluation, including attempts to circumvent the safety features.
- Conduct follow-up and obtain informal feedback; identify problems, and offer additional guidance.
- Monitor the use of the device to determine whether additional training is necessary or for any possible adverse effects of the device on patient care.

Your employer must document consideration and implementation of appropriate commercially available and effective engineering controls designed to eliminate or minimize exposure.

Many different evaluation forms can be used. The employer should maintain a file of the forms after they are completed with the action taken regarding the device.

Both active and passive safety features are available in safe needle systems. An integrated system is preferable because the safety feature is built in and is not dependent on employee compliance. **Table 3-1** lists the engineering features for devices designed to prevent sharps injury.

FYI

Self-Sheathing Needle Products
Even after activation, self-sheathing needle products and other SESIPs must be disposed of in a sharps container that conforms to the requirements of the standard.

Table 3-1 Engineering Features for Devices Designed to Prevent Sharps Injury

- A fixed safety feature provides a barrier between the hands and the needle after use; the safety feature should allow or require the worker's hands to remain behind the needle at all times.
- The safety feature is an integral part of the device, not an accessory.
- The safety feature is in effect before disassembly and remains in effect after disposal to protect users and trash handlers, and for environmental safety.
- The safety feature is as simple as possible and requires little or no training to use effectively.

OSHA Tips   CALIFORNIA

CalOSHA's regulation requires that hospitals, physicians, and other health care providers switch to safe needle systems.

In Case of Injury

According to the National Institute of Occupational Safety and Health, an estimated 600,000 needlestick injuries occur annually in the hospital setting. Hospital studies reveal that one third of all sharps injuries are related to the disposal process of the sharps.

If you are stuck by a needle containing blood or OPIMs, OSHA recommends the following:

- An HIV test and counseling
- A test for HIV periodically for at least 6 months
- Practice "safe" sex
- Stop breastfeeding
- Get immediate evaluation of any illness

You can also call the Needlestick Hotline (National Clinicians Postexposure Prophylaxis Hotline), which is run by the Department of Health and Human Services and which offers up-to-date, free advice in an emergency: (888) 448-4911.

Contaminated Sharps

OSHA defines contaminated sharps as any contaminated object that can penetrate the skin, including, but not limited to, needles, scalpels, broken capillary tubes, and exposed ends of dental wires **Figure 3-4**.

Contaminated needles or other contaminated sharps must not be bent, recapped, or removed unless it can be demonstrated that no alternative is feasible or that such action is required by a specific medical procedure.

If a procedure requires shearing or breaking of needles, this procedure must be specified in the company's exposure control plan. An acceptable means of demonstrating that no alternative to bending, recapping, or removing contaminated needles is feasible or that such action is required by a specific medical procedure would be a written justification (supported by reliable evidence). This also needs to be included as part of the exposure control plan. The justification must state the basis for the determination that no alternative is feasible or must specify that a particular medical procedure requires, for example, the bending of the needle and the use of forceps to accomplish this.

Needle removal or recapping needles must be accomplished through a one-handed technique or the use of a mechanical device **Skill Drill 3-1**:

1. Remove and recap needles through the use of a mechanical device or one-handed technique to prevent puncture wounds (**Step ❶**).
2. Using one hand, gently slide the needle into the needle cover (**Step ❷**).
3. Press the tip of the needle against the wall for support. Apply gentle pressure to secure the needle cover (**Step ❸**).

Nurses (RNs and LPNs) were injured more often than any other type of health care worker. An overwhelming majority (93%) of the injuries were caused by needles that did not have a safe design. The needles were not shielded, recessed, or retractable.

Reusable Sharps

Reusable sharps must be placed in clearly labeled, puncture-resistant, leak-proof containers immediately or as soon as possible after use until they can be reprocessed. The containers for reusable sharps are not required to be closable because it is anticipated that containers used for collecting and holding reusable sharps will be reused.

Reusable sharps, including pointed scissors that have been contaminated, must be decontaminated before reuse. Before cleaning, store the sharps in a container with a wide opening, and encourage people to use care in removing items.

Proper decontamination requires all visible blood or OPIMs to be rinsed off. Large amounts of organic debris interfere with the efficacy of the disinfecting/sterilization process.

Use a mechanical means (forceps or tongs) to remove contaminated sharps from containers; never reach into any container containing contaminated sharps with your hands. For example, employees must not reach into sinks filled with soapy water into which sharp instruments have been placed; appropriate controls in such a circumstance would include the use of strainer-type baskets to hold the instruments and forceps to remove and immerse the items **Figure 3-5**.

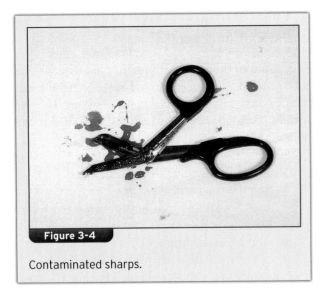

Figure 3-4

Contaminated sharps.

skill drill

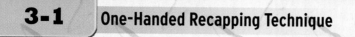

3-1   One-Handed Recapping Technique

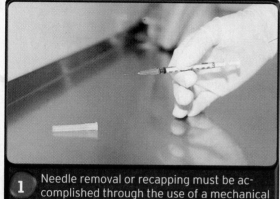

1 Needle removal or recapping must be accomplished through the use of a mechanical device or one-handed technique to prevent puncture wounds.

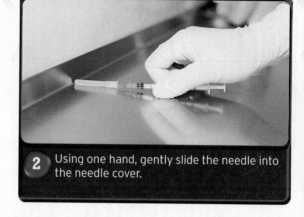

2 Using one hand, gently slide the needle into the needle cover.

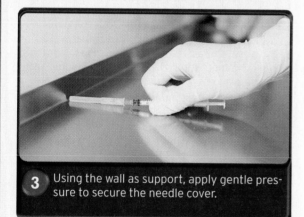

3 Using the wall as support, apply gentle pressure to secure the needle cover.

When it is necessary to examine the contents of a container, pour the contents of the container out onto a surface for inspection. An example is inspecting a bag for illegal drugs that might contain a contaminated needle or syringe. The intent is to provide conditions in which the contents can be seen and safely handled.

Acceptable Sharps Containers

The Food and Drug Administration regulates sharps disposal containers as Class II medical devices. OSHA's bloodborne pathogens standard establishes minimum design performance elements for sharps disposal containers. According to the standard, a sharps container must meet four criteria to be considered acceptable. It must be closable, puncture resistant, leakproof on sides and bottom, and labeled or color coded in accordance with the standard **Figure 3-6**.

A sharps container may be made of a variety of products, including cardboard or plastic, as long as the four criteria are met. Duct tape may be used to secure a sharps container lid, but it is not acceptable if it serves as the lid itself.

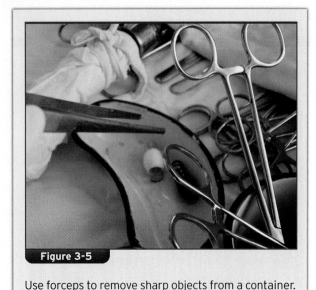

Figure 3-5

Use forceps to remove sharp objects from a container.

FYI

Food and Drug Administration Classification of Medical Devices

Class I devices (such as tongue depressors) are subject only to general regulatory controls and receive little agency oversight.

Class II devices (such as infant incubators) are subject to special controls, such as performance standards, to ensure their safe and effective use.

Class III devices (such as implantable pacemakers) are generally life sustaining or life supporting and are implanted in the body; they present an unreasonable risk of illness of injury.

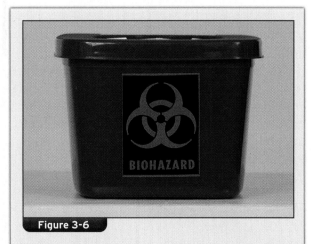

Figure 3-6

Biohazard symbols must be fluorescent orange or orange-red with letters or symbols in a contrasting color. These are attached to any container that is used to store or transport potentially infectious materials.

FYI

National Institute of Occupational Safety and Health Criteria for Safety Performance of Sharps Containers

1. Functionality: Containers should remain functional during their entire use. They should be durable, closable, leak resistant on their sides and bottoms, and puncture resistant until final disposal. A sufficient number of sharps disposal containers should be provided. Individual containers should have adequate volume and safe access to the disposal opening.

2. Accessibility: Containers should be accessible to workers who use, maintain, or dispose of sharp devices. Containers should be conveniently placed and (if necessary) portable within the workplace.

3. Visibility: Containers should be plainly visible to the workers who use them. Workers should be able to see the degree to which the container is full, proper warning labels, and color coding.

4. Accommodation: Container designs should be accommodating or convenient for the user and the facility, and they should be environmentally sound (eg, free of heavy metals and composed of recycled materials). Accommodation also includes ease of storage and assembly and simplicity of operation.

A sharps container must have a warning label affixed to it. The standard requires that warning labels "be affixed to containers of regulated waste, refrigerators and freezers containing blood or other potentially infectious material; and other containers used to store, transport, or ship blood or other potentially infectious materials."

Using Sharps Containers

Contaminated sharps must be discarded immediately or as soon as feasible into an acceptable sharps container.

Sharps containers must be easily accessible to personnel and located as close as feasible to the immediate area where sharps are used or can be reasonably anticipated to be found. Sharps containers mounted onto walls should be 52 to 56 inches from the floor.

Sharps containers must be maintained upright throughout use, routinely replaced, and not overfilled.

The replacement schedule must be clearly outlined in the exposure control plan. When contaminated sharps are being moved from the area of use, the container must be closed immediately before removal or replacement to prevent spillage or protrusion of contents during handling, storage, transport, or shipping.

If leakage is possible or if the outside of the container has become contaminated, the sharps container must be placed in a secondary container that is closable and constructed to contain all contents and prevent leakage during handling, storage, transport, or shipping.

Areas such as correctional facilities, psychiatric units, or pediatric units may have difficulty placing sharps containers in the immediate use area. If workers in these units use a mobile cart to hold the sharps container, it is necessary to lock the sharps container to the cart.

Laundries that handle contaminated laundry must have sharps containers easily accessible because of the incidence of needles mixed with laundry.

Facilities that handle shipments of waste that may contain contaminated sharps must also have sharps containers easily accessible in the event a package accidentally opens and releases sharps. All containers must be appropriately labeled with the owner of the container and their address.

The standard requires that reusable containers (such as those used to transport contaminated sharps for cleaning) not be opened, emptied, or cleaned manually or in any other manner that would expose employees to the risk of percutaneous injury. Finally, it is important to remember that whatever goes into a disposable sharps container *stays* in the sharps container. At no time is anyone allowed to go into a disposable sharps container. In many states, there are significant fines for anyone who tries to or goes into a disposable sharps container.

FYI

Needle Sheaths

A needle sheath of a self-sheathing needle is not to be considered a "waste container." A self-sheathing needle must be disposed of in a sharps container.

▶ Work Practice Controls

Work practice controls are the behaviors necessary to use engineering controls effectively. These include, but are not limited to, using sharps containers, using an eye-wash station, and washing your hands after removing PPE. An example of a work practice control would be to immediately place contaminated sharps into a sharps container.

All procedures involving blood or OPIMs must be performed in a manner that minimizes or eliminates splashing, spraying, splattering, and generation of droplets of these substances. Not only does this decrease the chances of direct exposure through spraying or splashing of infectious materials onto you, but it also reduces contamination of surfaces in the general work area.

Work practice controls must be evaluated and updated on a regular schedule to ensure their effectiveness.

Mouth pipetting or suctioning of blood or OPIMs is prohibited. This procedure should never occur unless it is part of a specialized procedure such as DeLee suctioning; however, even then there must be a one-way valve between the patient and the practitioner.

Eating, drinking, smoking, applying cosmetics or lip balm, and handling contact lenses are prohibited in work areas where there is a reasonable likelihood of occupational exposure to blood or OPIMs.

Employees are permitted to eat and drink in an ambulance cab, for example, as long as the employer has implemented procedures to permit employees to wash up and change contaminated clothing before entering the ambulance cab and to ensure that patients and contaminated material remain behind the separating partition.

Hand cream is not considered a cosmetic and is permitted under the standard; however, some petroleum-based hand creams can adversely affect glove integrity.

Food or drink must not be kept in refrigerators, freezers, shelves, cabinets, countertops, or benches where blood or OPIMs are present.

You must remove all PPE and wash your hands before leaving the work area. To prevent contamination of employee eating areas, you should not enter eating or break areas while wearing PPE **Figure 3-7** .

Handwashing and Handwashing Facilities

Handwashing is one of the most effective methods of preventing transmission of bloodborne pathogens. It is required that you wash your hands after removal of gloves and other PPE **Figure 3-8** .

FYI

Waterless Handwashing Systems
OSHA states that if there has been no occupational exposure to or contact with blood or OPIMs (as defined in the standard), the use of alcohol-based swabs described in the CDC's October 2002 guidelines would be appropriate.

Employers are required to provide handwashing facilities that are readily accessible to all employees. The standard specifies that the handwashing facility must be situated so that you do not have to use stairs, doorways, and corridors, which might result in environmental surface contamination.

When the provision of handwashing facilities is not feasible (such as in an ambulance or police car), the employer must provide either an appropriate antiseptic hand cleanser with clean cloth or paper towels or antiseptic towelettes. If you use antiseptic hand cleansers or towelettes, you must wash your hands (or other affected area) with soap and warm water as soon as possible after contact with blood or OPIMs **Figure 3-9** .

Employers must ensure you wash your hands, and any other contaminated skin, with soap and at least tepid running warm water (or flush mucous membranes with water) as soon as possible after

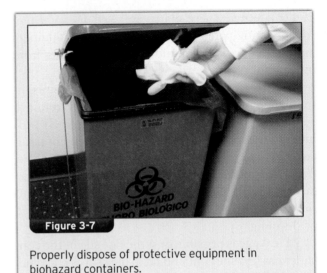
Figure 3-7
Properly dispose of protective equipment in biohazard containers.

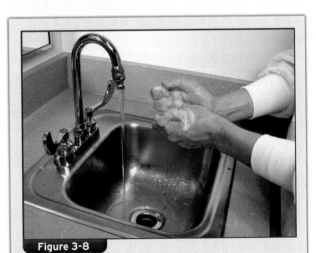
Figure 3-8
Handwashing is a primary means of preventing transmission of bloodborne pathogens.

contact with blood or OPIMs. Groups that may need to use alternative washing methods such as antiseptic hand cleansers and towelettes are ambulance-based EMTs, fire fighters, police, and mobile blood collection personnel.

Handwashing is required after the removal of gloves because although gloves (vinyl or latex) form a barrier they are not completely impermeable.

Cleaning Work Surfaces

The term *work area* means the area where work involving exposure or potential exposure to blood or

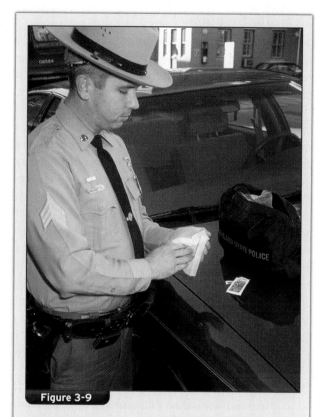

Figure 3-9

Antiseptic wipes can be used when handwashing is not an option.

FYI

Handwashing and Cleaning Work Surfaces

• There is no requirement for handwashing upon leaving the work area unless contact with blood or OPIMs has occurred or if you have removed gloves or other PPE.

• Employees must wash hands and skin surfaces after the removal of gloves or other PPE.

• Although extraordinary attempts to disinfect or sterilize environmental surfaces such as walls or floors are rarely indicated, routine cleaning and removal of soil are required.

patient waiting area), type of surface (carpet versus hard floor), type of soil present (gross contamination versus minor splattering), and procedure and tasks performed (laboratory analysis versus patient care). The cleaning schedule must occur at least weekly or after completion of tasks or procedures, after contamination of surfaces, or at the end of a shift if there is a possibility of contamination.

FYI

Proper Device Operation

Surgical power tools, lasers, and electrocautery devices may generate aerosols as well as be a source for splashing and spattering. Some of these devices include labeling recommendations such as local exhaust ventilation. Your employer is responsible for ensuring appropriate operation of these devices, including proper training and use of the controls recommended by the manufacturer.

OPIMs exists, along with the potential contamination of surfaces.

The term *worksite* not only refers to permanent fixed facilities such as hospitals, dental/medical offices, or clinics, but also covers temporary nonfixed workplaces. Examples of such facilities include, but are not limited to, ambulances, bloodmobiles, temporary blood collection centers, and any other nonfixed worksites that have a reasonable possibility of becoming contaminated with blood or OPIMs.

Your employer will identify which work surfaces require inspection for contamination with blood or OPIMs and have regularly scheduled decontamination. This could include, but is not limited to, wastebaskets, exam tables, counters, floors, ambulance interiors, and police cars.

After a regular inspection and cleaning schedule is established, it will need to be followed. The schedule must consider location (exam room versus

Receptacles

All bins, pails, cans, and similar receptacles intended for reuse that have a reasonable likelihood for becoming contaminated with blood or OPIMs should be inspected and decontaminated on a regularly scheduled basis. These receptacles should be cleaned and decontaminated immediately or as soon as feasible upon visible contamination.

Protective Coverings

Protective coverings, such as plastic wrap, aluminum foil, or imperviously backed absorbent paper used to cover equipment and environmental surfaces, should be removed and replaced as soon as feasible when they become overtly contaminated or at the end of the work shift if they may have become contaminated during the shift.

Work Practices

Work surface decontamination should be performed at the end of the work shift if the work surface may have become contaminated since the last cleaning by, for example, setting down contaminated instruments or specimens on the work surface. This requirement is based on the existence of a contaminated work surface rather than a particular worksite location. It does not, for example, encompass desks or countertops that remain uncontaminated.

Where procedures are performed on a continual basis throughout a shift or a day, as may be the case with a clinical laboratory technician performing blood analyses, it is not necessary for the work surface to be decontaminated before the technician can proceed to the next analysis. Rather, the contaminated work surfaces must be decontaminated after the procedures are completed (in this example, a set of analyses). The completion of procedures might also occur when the employee is going to leave the work area for a period of time.

> **FYI**
>
> **Cleaning Grossly Contaminated Surfaces**
> Whenever there is obvious contamination of a surface, first clean with a soap and water solution to ensure that the disinfectant is completely effective.

While cleaning up potentially infectious materials, you must wear disposable medical exam gloves and use an Environmental Protection Agency–approved solution. Follow the label instructions regarding the amount of disinfectant and the length of time it must remain wet on the surface. The effectiveness of a disinfectant is governed by strict adherence to the instructions on the label.

Cleansing Solutions

An example of an inexpensive approved solution is 10% bleach and water. Fresh solutions of diluted household bleach made up daily (every 24 hours) are also considered appropriate for disinfecting environmental surfaces and for decontamination of sites following initial cleanup of spills of blood or OPIMs. You should use disposable towels to clean up the spill and then dispose of the towels in a biohazard-labeled bag.

Do not clean up with your hands any broken glass that may be contaminated. Instead, use a dustpan and brush, cardboard, or tongs **Skill Drill 3-2**. The tools used in cleanup (such as forceps) must be properly decontaminated or discarded after use. Contaminated broken glass must be placed in a biohazard sharps container. Placing broken glass in a plastic bag may put others at risk for an occupational exposure incident. You must be given specific information and training with respect to this task.

1. When cleaning up broken glass, wear gloves and/or other PPE (**Step ❶**).
2. Do not clean up broken glass with your hands. Instead use a dust pan and brush, cardboard, or tongs (**Step ❷**).
3. Broken glass must be placed in an appropriate sharps container. Placing broken glass in plastic bag may put others at risk for exposure (**Steps ❸a** and **❸b**).

> **FYI**
>
> **Decontamination Issues**
> Decontamination is not automatically required after each procedure, but is required after procedures that result in surface contamination. There may be some instances in which "immediate" decontamination of overt contamination and spills may not be practical. More stringent decontamination rules, such as cleaning equipment or changing coverings between patients, may be prudent infection control policy but do not fall under OSHA's mandate to safeguard employee (not patient) health.

> **CAUTION**
>
> - HBV is able to survive for at least a week in dried blood on environmental surfaces or contaminated instruments.
> - Vacuum cleaners are prohibited for the cleaning of broken glass under the standard.

skill drill

3-2 Cleaning a Contaminated Spill

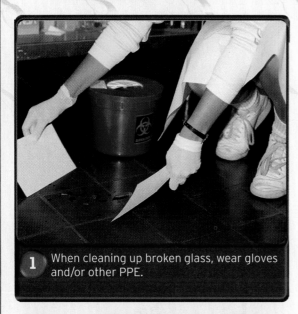

1 When cleaning up broken glass, wear gloves and/or other PPE.

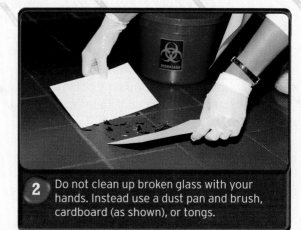

2 Do not clean up broken glass with your hands. Instead use a dust pan and brush, cardboard (as shown), or tongs.

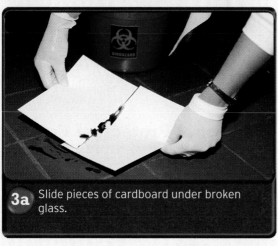

3a Slide pieces of cardboard under broken glass.

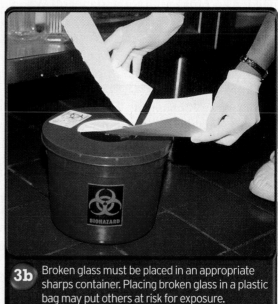

3b Broken glass must be placed in an appropriate sharps container. Placing broken glass in a plastic bag may put others at risk for exposure.

Laundry

Contaminated laundry should be sent to a facility following the OSHA standard. Your employer must determine whether the facility to which laundry is shipped uses universal precautions when handling all laundry. If not, all bags or containers of contaminated laundry must be labeled or color coded. Because red bags can indicate materials for disposal, many agencies use yellow bags with the biohazard symbol affixed to them to avoid confusion. The biohazard symbol must be affixed to any biohazard waste or contaminated materials such as laundry.

Do not handle laundry any more than necessary. Reducing the amount of manual handling of contaminated laundry reduces the risk of exposure to blood or OPIMs and will also reduce contamination of work surfaces in the laundry area.

Contaminated laundry should be bagged or placed in an approved container at the location where it was used and should not be sorted or rinsed in the location of use.

Contaminated laundry should be placed and transported in bags or containers labeled or color coded in accordance with the standard. When a facility uses universal precautions in the handling of all soiled laundry, alternative labeling or color coding is sufficient if it permits all employees to recognize that universal precautions are required in handling the containers **Figure 3-10** .

Whenever contaminated laundry is wet and presents a reasonable likelihood of soaking through or leaking from the bag or container, the laundry should be placed and transported in bags or containers that prevent soak-through and/or leakage of fluids to the exterior.

You must wear protective gloves (eg, utility gloves) and any other appropriate PPE to prevent or reduce contact exposure to blood or OPIMs when handling laundry or waste materials.

> **CAUTION**
>
> Home laundering of PPE is strictly prohibited. Current recommendations for the laundering of contaminated linen stipulate only that normal laundering methods are used according to the manufacturer's recommendations.

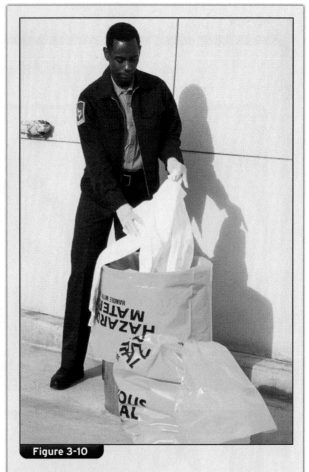

Figure 3-10

Contaminated laundry should be clearly labeled and placed in leak-proof containers.

Personal Protective Equipment

PPE is specialized clothing or equipment worn or used by you for protection against hazard. This includes equipment such as latex or vinyl gloves, gowns, aprons, face shields, masks, eye protection, laboratory coats, CPR microshields, and resuscitation bags. PPE prevents blood or OPIMs from passing through to or contacting your work or street clothes, undergarments, skin, eyes, mouth, or other mucous membranes **Figure 3-11** .

Resuscitator devices must be readily available and accessible to employees who can reasonably be expected to perform resuscitation procedures. Emergency ventilation devices also fall under the scope of PPE and therefore must be provided by the employer for use in resuscitation. This includes masks, mouthpieces, resuscitation bags, and shields/overlay barriers **Figure 3-12** .

CAUTION

DO NOT use a resuscitator device improperly. It is a violation of the standard.

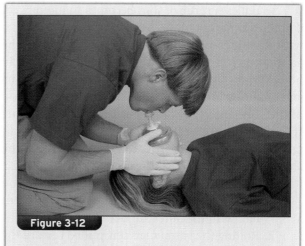

Figure 3-12

Using a pocket mask during CPR prevents exposure to potentially infectious body fluids.

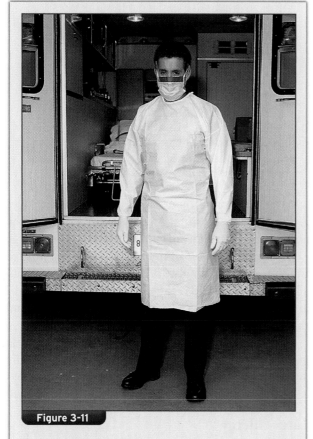

Figure 3-11

Full PPE includes gloves, gown, mask, and eye shield.

Reasonably anticipated spattering or generation of droplets would necessitate use of eye protection and mask or a face shield to prevent contamination of the mucous membranes of the eyes, nose, and mouth. Whenever you need to wear a face mask, you must also wear eye protection. If you are wearing your personal glasses, you must use side shields and plan to decontaminate your glasses and side shields according to the schedule determined by your employer.

PPE is acceptable if it prevents blood or OPIMs from contaminating work clothes, street clothes, un-dergarments, skin, eyes, mouth, or other mucous membranes. You must use PPE such as gloves or a mask whenever you might be exposed to blood or OPIMs.

Your employer is responsible for providing PPE at no expense to you. PPE must be provided in appropriate sizes and placed within easy reach for all employees. Your employer must evaluate the task and the type of exposure expected and, based on the determination, select the "appropriate" personal protective clothing. For example, laboratory coats or gowns with long sleeves must be used for procedures in which exposure of the forearm to blood or OPIMs is reasonably anticipated to occur.

Laboratory coats and uniforms that are used as PPE must be laundered by the employer and not sent home with the employee for cleaning. Although many employees have traditionally provided and laundered their own uniforms or laboratory coats if the item's intended function is to act as PPE, it is your employer's responsibility to provide, clean, repair, replace, and/or dispose of it.

It is necessary for you to be trained in the proper use of PPE. Report to your supervisor when any equipment is not available (such as a missing protective shield) or not in working order (such as a hole in an apron).

If blood or OPIMs contaminate your clothing, you must remove them as soon as feasible and place them in an appropriately designated area or container.

If a pullover scrub or shirt becomes contaminated, you must remove it in such a way as to avoid contact with the outer surface—for example, rolling up the garment as it is pulled toward the head for removal; however, if the blood penetrates the scrub or shirt and contaminates the inner surface, the penetration of the garment itself would constitute an exposure. If the scrub or shirt cannot be removed without contamination of the face, it is recommended that the shirt be cut and removed **Skill Drill 3-3** .

1. If a pullover shirt becomes contaminated, you must remove it in such a way as to avoid contact with the outer surface (**Step ❶**).
2. Rolling the garment as it is pulled toward the head will decrease the chance of contact with the contaminated area (**Step ❷**).
3. After rolling up the shirt, carefully pull it over the head to avoid contact with the face or mucous membranes (**Step ❸**).
4. If the shirt cannot be removed without contamination, it is recommended that the shirt be cut off (**Step ❹**).

If blood or OPIMs have penetrated your PPE, it is recommended that you check your body for cuts or scrapes or other nonintact skin when removing your equipment. The penetration itself would constitute an exposure of the skin.

You must remove all PPE before leaving the work area to prevent transmission of bloodborne pathogens to coworkers in other departments and family and to prevent contamination of environmental surfaces.

Gloves

Gloves must be used where there is reasonable anticipation of employee hand contact with blood, OPIMs, mucous membranes, or nonintact skin; when performing vascular access procedures; or when handling or touching contaminated surfaces or items.

Gloves are not necessary when administering intramuscular or subcutaneous injections as long as bleeding that could result in hand contact with blood or OPIMs is not anticipated. Gloves are not necessary when blood or OPIMs are not present or do not have the possibility of occurring.

FYI

Gloves
- Studies have shown that gloves provide a barrier, but that neither vinyl nor latex procedure gloves are completely impermeable.
- Disinfecting agents may cause deterioration of the glove material; washing with surfactants could result in wicking or enhanced penetration of liquids into the glove via undetected pores, thereby transporting blood and OPIMs into contact with the hand. For this reason, disposable (single-use) gloves may not be washed and reused.
- Certain solutions such as iodine may cause discoloration of gloves without affecting their integrity and function.

It is important to consider that the use of gloves is required for any situation that might reasonably be anticipated to result in an exposure to blood or OPIMs. For example, the use of pneumatic tube systems for the transport of laboratory specimens requires that all employees should regard the contents as hazardous and must wear gloves when removing specimens from the tube system carrier.

Hypoallergenic gloves, glove liners, powderless gloves, or other similar alternatives must be readily available and accessible at no cost to those employees who are allergic to the gloves normally provided.

Latex Allergy

Natural rubber latex (NRL) is a glove material that has been used in the health care environment for barrier protection for many years. In response to reported

CAUTION

Whenever clothing is blood soaked, the employee must be permitted to change into fresh garments before continuing with work. A paramedic on an emergency call whose garments become blood soaked but continues to the next call without a change of clothing would be in violation of the standard.

skill drill

3-3   Removing Contaminated Equipment

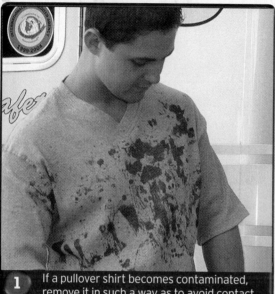

1 If a pullover shirt becomes contaminated, remove it in such a way as to avoid contact with the outer surface.

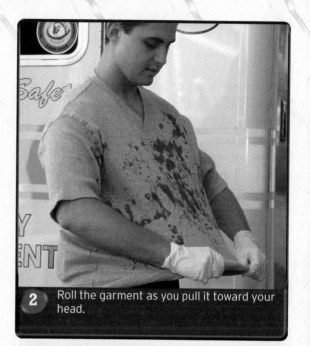

2 Roll the garment as you pull it toward your head.

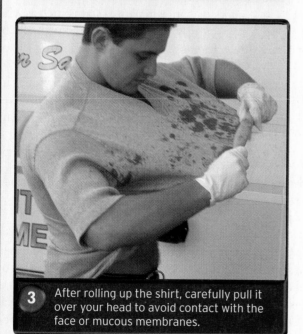

3 After rolling up the shirt, carefully pull it over your head to avoid contact with the face or mucous membranes.

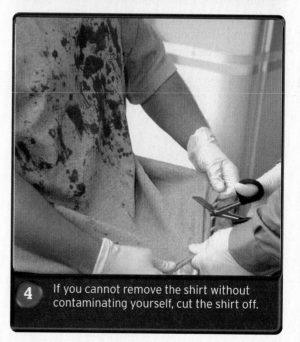

4 If you cannot remove the shirt without contaminating yourself, cut the shirt off.

NRL allergy in some patients and health care workers, new measures have been recommended to reduce the risk of NRL allergy in workers.

The signs and symptoms of latex allergies include rashes, inflammation (immediate or delayed), respiratory irritation, asthma, and in rare cases, shock.

The groups that fall in the high-risk category for latex allergies include health care workers and workers in the latex industry.

Latex cross-reacts with allergies to certain foods such as avocados, apricots, bananas (most frequent reaction), chestnuts, grapes, kiwi, passion fruit, pears, and pineapples.

The occupational issues with latex allergies include more than just the affected employee. Workers with latex sensitivities must use nonlatex gloves, and their coworkers must use either nonpowdered latex or nonlatex gloves.

Sources of latex exposure can be separated into two categories: medical and household. The possible latex exposures in each of these categories are as follows:

Medical: Gloves, urinary catheters, face masks, tourniquet, adhesive tape, bandages, wound drains, injection ports, electrode pads, rubber syringe stoppers and medication vial stoppers, bulb syringes, mattresses on stretchers, dental devices, stethoscopes and blood pressure cuff tubing, resuscitation bags, PCA syringes, and dental dams.
Effective September 30, 1998, the Food and Drug Administration requires labeling statements for medical devices that contain NRL and prohibits the use of the word "hypoallergenic" to describe such products.
Household: Balloons, condoms or diaphragms, rubber bands, shoe soles, erasers, toys, sports equipment **Figure 3-13**, carpet backing, feeding nipples or pacifiers, elastic on underwear, food handled with powdered latex gloves, handles on racquets, tools, diapers, sanitary and incontinence pads, computer mouse pads, and buttons on electronic equipment.

Limited Exceptions to Using PPE

There are a few exceptions to the use of PPE when the use of such equipment would prevent the proper delivery of health care or public safety services or

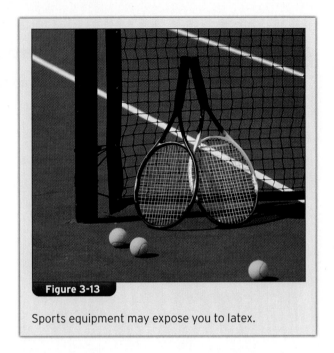

Figure 3-13

Sports equipment may expose you to latex.

would pose an increased hazard to the personal safety of the worker. Examples of such situations could include the following:

- A sudden change in patient status such as when an apparently stable patient unexpectedly begins to hemorrhage profusely, putting the patient's life in immediate jeopardy.
- A fire fighter rescuing an individual who is not breathing from a burning building discovers that the resuscitation equipment is lost or damaged and must administer CPR.
- A bleeding person unexpectedly attacks a police officer with a knife, threatening the safety of the officer and/or coworkers.

▶ Universal Precautions

Universal precautions is an aggressive, standardized approach to infection control. According to the concept of universal precautions, you should treat all human blood and certain body fluids as if they are known to contain HIV, HBV, HCV, or other blood-borne pathogens, regardless of the perceived risk of the source. Examples of incidents that do and do not required universal precautions are included in **Table 3-2** .

Materials That Require Universal Precautions

Universal precautions apply to the following potentially infectious materials:
- Blood
- Semen
- Vaginal secretions
- Cerebrospinal fluid
- Synovial fluid
- Pleural fluid
- Any body fluid with visible blood
- Any unidentifiable body fluid
- Saliva from dental procedures

Materials That Do Not Require Universal Precautions

Universal precautions do not apply to the following body fluids unless they contain visible blood:
- Feces
- Nasal secretions
- Sputum

- Sweat
- Tears
- Urine
- Vomitus

CAUTION

Food-handling gloves are not appropriate as PPE because they fail to meet the requirements of the standard.

▶ Body Substance Isolation

Another method of infection control is called <u>body substance isolation (BSI)</u>. This method defines *all* body fluids and substances as infectious. BSI includes not only the fluids and other materials covered by this standard, but also expands coverage to all body fluids and substances.

BSI is an acceptable alternative to universal precautions provided facilities using BSI adhere to all other provisions of this standard.

Table 3-2 Determining the Need for Universal Precautions

Incident	Universal Precautions Needed?	Suggested Action
Nurse is going to change dressing on a recent wound.	Yes	Nurse should wear latex or vinyl gloves and/or PPE whenever at risk of exposure to blood or potentially infectious materials.
Teacher is approached by young, hysterical student with a bloody nose.	Yes	If required to attend to the student, the teacher should reassure child, put on latex or vinyl gloves, and follow routine procedures.
A neighbor is called to a home where an older man appears to have had a heart attack. The man is conscious and able to speak.	No	There is no immediate blood or infectious materials, although the neighbor may need to perform CPR in the event of cardiac or respiratory arrest. *Note:* In the event of cardiac or respiratory arrest, work practice controls and PPE may be required.
A police officer pulls over a car that has a burned-out headlight.	No	It is unlikely that the police officer will come in contact with blood or potentially infectious materials.
A laboratory worker is testing urine for evidence of infection. The specimen appears to have a trace of blood.	Yes	The laboratory worker should be using PPE whenever dealing with any specimens with visible blood.

Site-Specific Work Page

Employee Training

1. Labeling methods at this worksite include the following:

   Color: _____

   Biohazard symbol (label): _____

   Words: _____

   Red bag: _____

2. The person to notify if you discover regulated waste containers, refrigerators containing blood or OPIMs, or contaminated equipment without proper labels is: _____

3. At my worksite, we are expected to adhere to the concept of universal precautions: ☐ True   ☐ False

4. According to my employer's exposure control plan, sharps containers are to be inspected every _____ and replaced when _____

   _____

5. Three examples of engineering controls at my worksite are:

   _____

   _____

   _____

   _____

   _____

6. The handwashing station nearest to my worksite is located at:

   _____

   _____

▶ Vital Vocabulary

<u>body substance isolation (BSI)</u> Defines all body fluids and substances as infectious.

<u>clinical laboratory</u> A workplace where diagnostic or other screening procedures are performed on blood or other potentially infectious materials.

<u>universal precautions</u> An approach to infection control. According to the concept of Universal Precautions, all human blood and certain human body fluids are treated as if known to be infectious for HIV, HBV, HCV, and other bloodborne pathogens.

<u>work area</u> The area where work involving exposure or potential exposure to blood or OPIM exists, along with the potential contamination of surfaces.

▶ Check Your Knowledge

1. A gown that is frequently ripped or falls apart under normal use would be considered "appropriate PPE."
   A. True
   B. False

2. The exposure control plan describes the engineering controls in use at a worksite.
   A. True
   B. False

3. Duct tape may be used to secure a sharps container lid.
   A. True
   B. False

4. When cleaning up potentially contaminated broken glass, you may use a dust pan and brush, cardboard, or an industrial vacuum cleaner.
   A. True
   B. False

5. You may launder your own PPE, but only if this is clearly specified in the exposure control plan.
   A. True
   B. False

6. Gloves must be used where there is reasonable anticipation of employee hand contact with blood.
   A. True
   B. False

7. Your employer must supply hypo-allergenic gloves at no cost to employees who are allergic to the gloves normally provided.
   A. True
   B. False

8. Containers of contaminated laundry do not need to be labeled.
   A. True
   B. False

9. Universal precautions do not apply to sweat or tears unless they contain visible blood.
   A. True
   B. False

10. Handwashing is not required after the removal of gloves.
    A. True
    B. False

Answers: 1. B; 2. A; 3. A; 4. B; 5. B; 6. A; 7. A; 8. B; 9. A; 10. B

Exposure Control Plan

▶ What Is an Exposure Control Plan?

The exposure control plan exists as a guideline for employees to know what to do when an exposure occurs. You do not have time to determine what to do *during* an exposure event. A well-documented exposure control plan resolves most of the questions that might arise about an exposure. In addition, the exposure control plan is a key provision of the Occupational Safety and Health Administration (OSHA) Bloodborne Pathogens Standard. A requirement of the plan is for the employer to identify the individuals who should receive training, protective equipment, vaccination, and other protections of the standard.

The plan must be reviewed annually and updated to reflect significant modifications in tasks or procedures that may result in occupational exposure to blood or other potentially infectious materials (OPIMs). The plan cannot offer protection to employees if it is filed away as soon as it is written and never reviewed again. It is also important that all employees who fall under the guidance of the plan be trained according to the plan **Figure 4-1** .

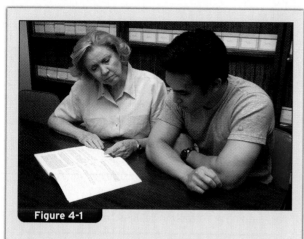

Figure 4-1

All employees must be made aware of an employer's exposure control plan.

A hard copy of the exposure control plan must be made available to an employee within 15 working days of his or her request. A sample exposure control plan is included in Appendix C. Please refer to it for guidance relative to compliance with OSHA's Bloodborne Pathogens Standard.

▶ Exposure Control Plan Requirements

According to OSHA, the exposure control plan should contain an exposure determination, including the following:

- *The exposure determination*: Each employer must determine which employees potentially have an occupational exposure to blood or OPIMs. This determination is made by reviewing job descriptions to see which employees could be exposed to blood or OPIMs on the job. The employer has to create the list of all tasks and procedures where occupational exposure could occur. This exposure determination has to be made without regard to the use of personal protective equipment.
- The schedule and method of implementation for each of the applicable subsections:
  - Methods of compliance
  - HIV, hepatitis B virus, and hepatitis C virus research laboratories and <u>production facilities</u>

  - Hepatitis B vaccination and postexposure evaluation and follow-up
  - Communication of hazards to employees
  - Record keeping of this standard
- Each employer needs to ensure that a copy of the exposure control plan is accessible to employees in accordance with 29 CFR 1910.1020(e).
- The exposure control plan is required to be reviewed and updated at least annually and whenever necessary to reflect new or modified tasks and procedures that affect occupational exposure and to reflect new or revised employee positions with occupational exposure. The review and update of such plans also need to do the following:
  - Reflect changes in technology that eliminate or reduce exposure to bloodborne pathogens
  - Document annually consideration and implementation of appropriate commercially available and effective safer medical devices designed to eliminate or minimize occupational exposure

The exposure control plan must include the procedure for evaluating the circumstances surrounding exposure incidents **Figure 4-2** .

Any employer who is required to establish an exposure control plan also needs to solicit input from nonmanagerial employees responsible for direct patient care who are potentially exposed to injuries from contaminated sharps in the identification, evaluation, and selection of effective engineering and work practice controls and shall document the solicitation in the exposure control plan.

The exposure control plan needs to be made available to the assistant secretary and the director upon request for examination and copying.

FYI

Computer Access to the Exposure Control Plan

If the exposure control plan is maintained solely on computer, employees must be trained to operate the computer.

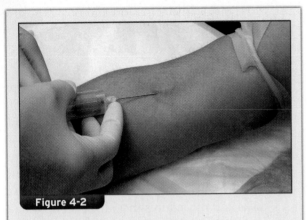

Figure 4-2

All procedures that risk occupational exposure must be outlined in the exposure control plan.

FYI

Reviewing and Updating the Plan

According to the preamble to the standard, the requirement to review and update the plan means that the plan must reflect changes in technology that eliminate or reduce exposure to bloodborne pathogens. The preamble to the Final Rule in 1991 also stated that "with regard to percutaneous incidents, such as needlestick injuries, evidence indicated that most injuries were preventable. . . . Seventy-five percent of all exposure incidents are caused by disposable syringes . . . and could be prevented by using syringes which incorporate resheathing or retracting designs."

OSHA Tips   CALIFORNIA

California OSHA adds the following requirements (effective August 1999):

- An effective procedure for gathering the information required by the sharps injury log
- An effective procedure for periodic determination of the frequency of use of the types and brands of sharps involved in the exposure incidents documented on the sharps injury log
- Frequency of use that may be approximated by any reasonable and effective method (eg, looking at purchase records or in-house tracking records)
- An effective procedure for identifying currently available engineering controls, and selecting such controls, where appropriate, for the procedures performed by employees in their respective work areas or departments

- An effective procedure for documenting patient safety determinations made pursuant to Exception 2, of subsection (d)(3)(A)
- An effective procedure for obtaining the active involvement of employees in reviewing and updating the exposure control plan with respect to the procedures performed by employees in their respective work areas or departments
- The exposure control plan shall be made available to the chief of the National Institute for Occupational Safety and Health or their respective designee upon request for examination and copying.

prep
kit

▶ Vital Vocabulary

<u>production facilities</u> Facilities engaged in industrial-scale, large-volume, or high-concentration production of HIV, HBV, or HCV.

▶ Check Your Knowledge

1. Exposure control plans are not necessary because you would have time to determine what to do during an exposure event.
   A. True
   B. False
2. An exposure control plan must be reviewed
   A. When there is adequate time
   B. Annually
   C. Only after an exposure
   D. If you have more than three exposures in a year
3. A hard copy of the plan must be made available to an employee who requests it within _____ days.
   A. 3
   B. 5
   C. 10
   D. 15

4. If the exposure control plan is maintained solely on computer, employees must be trained to operate the computer.
   A. True
   B. False
5. The exposure control plan must include the procedure for evaluating the circumstances surrounding exposure incidents.
   A. True
   B. False

Answers: 1. B; 2. B; 3. D; 4. A; 5. A

5

Common and Unusual Infectious Diseases

▶ Overview

This chapter describes some common and also some very unusual infectious diseases. The descriptions are not meant to be exhaustive, but rather focus on basic facts about common diseases that we see almost every day and those that we recognize because they are in the news. At the conclusion of this chapter, you should be able to:

- Identify symptoms associated with common infections.
- Explain differences in symptoms and illness caused by the same virus or bacteria.
- Describe unusual diseases that might be encountered because of international travel.
- Describe good handwashing habits.
- Explain the proper steps for using respiratory protections.

Air travel has allowed people to reach places all over the world. As more and more people travel, the risk of spreading serious infectious diseases increases. It is important to keep up-to-date on the various diseases and how to remain safe from the spread of these diseases.

Many of the diseases described in this chapter are well known to you and your family health care provider. Today, because of the development of new vaccines, diseases such as chicken pox, although not yet gone, are under much better control; however, new strains of bacteria are emerging that are increasingly resistant to some of our strongest antibiotic medications, as in the case of methicillin-resistant *Staphylococcus aureus* (MRSA). Although our success in eliminating the causes of serious illness and disease is mixed, we face a new challenge today. Terrorists may attempt to infect entire communities with deadly diseases. Hospital emergency department staff must prepare and practice steps necessary to diagnose, treat, and isolate rapidly potential victims of a terrorist attack using biological agents. In addition, the ease of international travel makes it more likely that an exotic or new illness could spread around the world in a matter of hours or days. The outbreak of severe acute respiratory syndrome (SARS), which first appeared in China in 2002, demonstrates how quickly one or two patients with an illness can affect countries all around the world in a very short time. Travelers who had no evidence of illness on departure developed symptoms soon after arriving at their destinations. In some cases, these patients unknowingly spread the infection to friends, family, and health care workers. Stopping the spread of infectious diseases requires high levels of suspicion and strong local, national, and international cooperation to mount a quick response to the sudden appearance of any unusual infectious disease.

▶ Chicken Pox

Chicken pox is a viral disease that is highly contagious. A person with chicken pox is contagious until the last blister has formed a scab. The disease is spread from person to person by direct contact or breathing in droplets released into the air by the infected person's coughing or sneezing. Most cases of chicken pox occur in children under 15 years of age, and the disease is most commonly seen in the spring. After the introduction of a vaccine, both the number of cases and the number of deaths caused by the disease declined.

Symptoms

Symptoms include:
- Fever
- Tiredness
- Itchy rash of blister-like sores

Serious complications include:
- Bacterial infection of the sores
- Pneumonia
- Encephalitis (swelling of the brain)

Diagnosis

The characteristic rash begins on the trunk and spreads out to the head, hands, and feet. The exam is very specific for the illness, and a detailed history helps to determine the source of the infection and who else might be at risk for the disease. Administration of the vaccine 3 to 5 days after exposure may modify the intensity of the disease. It is recommended that susceptible people be immunized within 3 days of exposure to a person with chicken pox.

Treatment

Scratching can cause blisters to become infected. Some relief from the itch of the blisters is possible. The use of lotions and oatmeal baths provides soothing relief.

FYI

Shingles

The chicken pox virus causes shingles. Cases of shingles have occurred as a result of vaccination, and these cases are seen in a younger population than those that occur after naturally occurring chicken pox. Shingles more commonly appear in people over 50 years of age.

Shingles causes numbness, itching, and severe pain, which are followed by a cluster of blisters that appear in a strip. This clustering of blisters reminds people of the shingles on the side of a house. Shingles may persist for months, and even if the rash resolves, persistent pain known as *postherpetic neuralgia* may occur.

Antiviral medication may be used to help treat the disease. Your health care provider determines whether the use of an antiviral medication or any other medication is required. Fever persisting for more than 4 days requires evaluation by a health care provider. It is important to avoid the use of aspirin for symptom relief. Use nonaspirin medications such as acetaminophen.

What Happens After Infection

Although unusual, some people are infected with the chicken pox virus more than once. For most people, the first infection will give lifelong immunity to the disease.

Prevention

Chicken pox may be prevented by vaccination.

▶ Group A Streptococcal Disease

Group A streptococcal disease (GAS) is a bacterium that is normally found on the skin and in the throats of healthy people. GAS is responsible for a variety of illnesses, which range from the common "strep" throat and impetigo (weeping infections of the skin) to life-threatening diseases such as necrotizing fasciitis, which has been sensationalized in the media as "flesh-eating bacteria."

Symptoms

Symptoms vary and include:
- No illness
- Fever
- Sore throat
- Swollen glands
- Rash
- Honey-crusted sores on the skin

Severe symptoms affecting skin wounds include:
- Fever

At the wound site:
- Severe pain
- Swelling
- Redness

In cases of streptococcal toxic shock syndrome:
- Fever
- Chills
- Muscle aches
- Rash (widely distributed over the body)
- Vomiting and diarrhea

Diagnosis

Diagnosis is determined by history, appearance of affected areas during physical exam, and a culture of material from the affected area.

FYI
Scarlet Fever
- Scarlet fever is caused by a particular strain of GAS and is associated with a sandpaper-like bumpy rash. There is a pale area around the lips, and the tongue is described as looking like a strawberry because of the white coating and red bumps.
- Skin around the toes and fingers may peel 7 to 10 days after the start of the infection.

FYI
Necrotizing Fasciitis
- It is caused by a variety of bacteria that grow in cuts or abrasions and release toxins.
- Necrotizing fasciitis destroys muscles, fat, and skin tissue.
- This disease can be rapidly progressive, which is why it receives so much attention from the media.

Treatment

Treatment with an appropriate antibiotic is indicated.

Prevention

Good handwashing and covering the mouth and nose when coughing and sneezing help to reduce the spread of the disease. Avoid sharing drinks, cups, and eating utensils.

Taking medication properly and completing the full course of treatment are especially important in controlling the spread of the bacteria. If infected wounds are not responding to standard treatment of cleansing and bandaging and the site becomes red, swollen, and painful, medical evaluation should be sought.

FYI

Streptococcal Toxic Shock Syndrome

- Streptococcal toxic shock syndrome causes the blood pressure to drop and major organs such as the liver and kidneys to fail.
- Symptoms include fever, rash, and low blood pressure.

▶ Hantavirus Pulmonary Syndrome

First recognized in 1993 in the southwest area of the United States, hantavirus pulmonary syndrome (HPS) is a deadly disease found throughout the United States. The source of the infection is contact with rodent droppings, urine, saliva, and nesting materials. Rarely is infection caused by the bite of an infected rodent. Only certain species of rodents (deer mice) are known to carry the disease. There is no known transmission by insect bites or from other animals.

The virus is primarily transmitted when people come into contact with contaminated air. Most often, contact occurs when people are cleaning infested areas. Sweeping, raking, or otherwise disturbing the area causes the dust containing the virus to float into the air. A person may breathe in the dust, touch something that is contaminated by the dust, and then wipe his or her nose or mouth or eat something that has become contaminated.

Any place that infected rodents nest, such as sheds, barns, warehouses, or summer cottages, may be a source of infection; therefore, it is important to avoid contact or take appropriate precautions when cleaning or working in or around areas potentially infested with rodents.

You cannot get the infection from touching, kissing, or caring for someone infected with HPS; the infection does not spread from person to person.

Symptoms

There have been only 363 cases of confirmed HPS in the United States. Because of the limited number of cases, the exact time from exposure to developing symptoms is not known. It is estimated that symptoms develop in 1 to 5 weeks.

Most frequent symptoms include:
- Fever
- Muscle ache
- Nausea
- Vomiting
- Cough

Other symptoms include:
- Dizziness
- Joint aches
- Shortness of breath

Diagnosis

The illness is very serious, and diagnosis is made by history of recent activity, physical exam, laboratory tests, and chest X-ray films. Confirmation of HPS is provided by specific blood tests.

Usually starting with a fever, the illness may lead to low blood pressure and failure of the liver and kidneys. The low blood pressure does not result in shock until the onset of respiratory failure due to fluid buildup in the lungs.

Treatment

Early aggressive treatment is necessary and may include intensive care unit monitoring to be sure that blood pressure is maintained and that airways and breathing are properly supported. The disease rapidly progresses, and 50% of patients infected with the disease may die.

Prevention

Control mice inside and outside. Use safety precautions. When it is necessary to work in areas that are currently or have been previously infested with rodents, follow these basic steps:
- Wear protective clothing such as coveralls and gloves.
- Do not sweep or vacuum mouse or rat droppings or nests, as this will cause the virus to go into the air.
- Spray the area and potentially infected materials (nesting, droppings, etc.) with a 10% solution of bleach or other disinfectant.
- Place the collected material into a plastic bag and seal the bag.
- Do not eat food in the affected area.
- Decontaminate clothing, and wash exposed areas after working in contaminated areas.

▶ Influenza

Influenza, or flu, is a viral illness that is easily spread from person to person. Epidemics of flu occur in late fall to early spring. Rates of infection with flu are highest for children and persons older than 65 years of age and anyone with health care problems that put them at greater risk for complications.

Symptoms

Symptoms associated with flu include
- Abrupt onset
- Fever
- Muscle aches
- Body aches
- Sore throat
- Runny nose
- Nonproductive cough

Diagnosis

Diagnostic tests are available for detection of flu virus infection. Rapid diagnostic tests allow health care providers to know whether a patient has the flu within 30 minutes.

Treatment

Treatment is symptomatic and may include early use of antiviral drugs. There are antiviral medications for treating the flu. Antiviral medications should be administered within 2 days of illness onset.

FYI

Lassa Fever
- First identified in 1969 in the town of Lassa, Nigeria, this virus is spread by mouse droppings, urine, and nesting materials.
- Found in portions of West Africa, each year 150,000 or more people are infected by the virus.
- Approximately 5,000 will die of the disease.
- A major complication of the disease is deafness.
- Up to one third of the people who recover will suffer permanent hearing loss.

Prevention

The best single method to prevent the flu is to get vaccinated each fall. Other methods include handwashing, covering your mouth and nose when sneezing or coughing, remaining at home when sick, and avoiding close contact with people who have cold or flu-like symptoms.

▶ Avian Influenza

Avian influenza, commonly known as "avian flu" or "bird flu," is caused by influenza type A viruses that normally only occur in birds. Avian flu is very contagious among birds and can cause some domesticated birds, such as chickens, ducks, and turkeys, to become very sick or die. These viruses usually do not infect humans, but in recent years, several cases of avian flu infection in humans have been reported.

There are several subtypes of avian influenza A viruses. The subtype that has become a major concern is the avian influenza A (H5N1) virus, which has caused the deaths of millions of birds and also poses a health risk to humans.

Symptoms

Symptoms associated with flu include:
- Fever
- Cough
- Sore throat
- Muscle aches

Symptoms may also include:
- Diarrhea
- Eye infections
- Pneumonia
- Severe respiratory diseases
- Other severe and life-threatening complications

Diagnosis

The symptoms of avian influenza may depend on which virus caused the infection but often are similar to those associated with human seasonal influenza.

Individuals with these symptoms may be experiencing an illness other than influenza; therefore, laboratory tests can be used to confirm avian influenza infection in humans.

FYI

Flu

- Each year in the United States, flu will result in approximately 36,000 deaths.
- Pandemics occur when many countries report widespread outbreak of the flu virus. This often results in significantly higher death rates. The outbreak of flu in 1918 is the best-known example of a pandemic. There are predictions that the avian flu could become the next pandemic flu and affect 33% of the population at one time, with up to 33% of these individuals succumbing to the disease.
- The collection of viral cultures is critical because the virus isolated from the culture provides specific information about influenza strains and subtypes. This information is used to guide formulation of vaccine for the next year.

Treatment

Prescription antiviral drugs approved for influenza (based on seasonal outbreak data) may be of some benefit in treating avian flu infection in humans; however, influenza viruses can become resistant to these drugs, and thus, these medications may not always work. For some of these drugs to be most effective, they must be taken within 48 hours after the first sign of symptoms.

Prevention

Use proper hand hygiene practices. Clean your hands often and thoroughly, preferably using soap and water for 15 to 20 seconds (or a waterless, alcohol-based hand rub when soap is not available), especially if you are handling poultry or poultry products.

If possible, avoid contact with poultry and other birds suspected or known to be infected. Avoid eating uncooked or undercooked poultry or poultry products. If you are sick, stay at home except to get medical attention. Cover your mouth and nose when you cough or sneeze.

▶ Legionellosis

Legionellosis is a disease caused by a bacterium. The disease has two forms: Legionnaire's disease, the most serious form, and Pontiac fever, the milder form.

Legionnaire's disease is caused by the inhalation of droplets containing the bacteria. These droplets may come from air-conditioning cooling towers, whirlpool spas, or showers contaminated by the bacteria. It is not spread person to person.

People at particular risk to develop Legionnaire's disease are those who smoke cigarettes, have chronic lung disease, or have a suppressed immune system. It takes about 2 to 10 days from exposure to develop the illness.

Pontiac fever, on the other hand, tends to strike healthy individuals, and symptoms develop within a few hours to 2 days from exposure to the bacteria.

Symptoms

The symptoms of Legionnaire's disease include:
- Fever
- Chills
- Cough
- Other flu-like symptoms
- Pneumonia

The symptoms of Pontiac fever include:
- Fever
- Muscle aches

Patients with this form of the disease do not experience pneumonia.

Diagnosis

Diagnosis requires a special test that is not routinely performed; therefore, the health care provider must take a careful history and be suspicious regarding possible exposure to the bacteria. Tests of sputum, urine, or blood will confirm diagnosis.

Treatment

Treatment is unnecessary for Pontiac fever. Legionnaire's disease is treated with antibiotics.

FYI

Legionnaire's Disease

- An estimated 8,000 to 18,000 people are infected with Legionnaire's disease in the United States each year.
- About 5% to 30% of people with Legionnaire's disease die.
- Outbreaks usually occur in the summer and early fall, but may occur any time of year.

What Happens After Infection

A major health care concern for patients with Legionnaire's disease is that they may develop life-threatening pneumonia.

Prevention

Improved design of air handling systems and the maintenance of cooling towers and plumbing systems are the main methods to prevent this disease.

▶ MRSA

Staph is one of the most common causes of skin infection in the United States but may cause different kinds of illness. It may cause bone infections, pneumonia, life-threatening blood infections, and other serious illnesses. Outbreaks of infections caused by MRSA have often been associated with health care institutions. MRSA is now appearing commonly in the community.

Transmission of MRSA usually occurs through close skin contact.

Symptoms

Symptoms commonly seen include:
- Weeping sores on the skin
- Boils
- Pimples

Diagnosis

Culture of the infection will lead to proper diagnosis.

Treatment

Simply draining the sore may be enough to cure the infection. Both general staph infections and infections caused by MRSA, however, respond to antibiotic treatment when necessary.

Prevention

Maintaining good hygiene and avoiding contact with drainage from skin lesions is the best method of prevention.

FYI

MRSA

- Participants in competitive sports may be at risk for MRSA infections. Risk factors include physical contact, skin damage, and sharing equipment or clothing.
- When participating in a sport, do not share towels or personal items, and inform the coach or trainer about any skin sores.
- Staph and MRSA often are found on the skin and in the nose of some people without causing illness; this is known as a carrier state and does not require treatment.

▶ West Nile Virus

First isolated in the West Nile district of Uganda in 1937, West Nile virus (WNV) has been recognized as a source of human illness in the eastern United States since 1999. The primary hosts for WNV are birds, particularly crows. Bird migration has resulted in WNV spreading quickly across the United States. Birds have not yet developed immunity to the disease.

Mosquitoes become infected from feeding on the blood of infected birds. The infected mosquitoes then transmit WNV to humans and other animals. Because mosquitoes are the source of transmission, the season for the disease begins in the spring, reaching its peak about mid August to September. Serious illness, such as encephalitis (inflammation of the brain) or meningitis (inflammation of the membrane around the brain and spinal cord), may result from infection. People over 50 years of age are at greatest risk for developing severe disease.

You cannot become infected from touching, kissing, or caring for someone who is infected with WNV; the infection does not spread from person to person. Detecting the presence of virus within any area is by dead bird–based surveillance. States gather data in areas where people report finding dead birds. Quantifying the intensity of the viral transmission within the area is determined by mosquito-based surveillance, which involves collecting mosquitoes and determining how many are infected.

Symptoms

The majority of infected people will have fever or no symptoms at all. Symptoms appear 2 to 15 days after being bitten by an infected mosquito. Symptoms, when they occur, are usually mild and may include:

- Fever
- Headache
- Muscle ache
- Backache
- Rash
- Swollen lymph nodes

The symptoms of more serious illness include:

- Tremor
- Stiff neck
- Severe headache
- Paralysis
- Muscle weakness
- Disorientation
- Convulsions
- Coma

Diagnosis

Diagnosis of the illness includes blood tests, a spinal tap (procedure to sample the fluid around the brain and spine), or magnetic resonance imaging.

Treatment

No specific treatment exists. Depending on the severity of the symptoms, hospitalization may be required. In most cases, a person will need to rest and take medication such as acetaminophen or other anti-inflammatory medication for headache and muscle aches. It is important to contact a health care provider if a temperature greater than 102°F (39°C) develops, or the headache is very severe or worsening or there are signs of the person acting confused or experiencing weakness.

What Happens After Infection

Most people will make a full recovery. Recovery from serious illness may take weeks. Those with more serious infections may suffer permanent injury to their nervous system. After recovering from infection, a person is immune to future WNV infection.

Prevention

To reduce mosquito breeding, routinely drain standing water in old tires, buckets, barrels, and flowerpots. When going outdoors, follow these precautions:

- Avoid times when mosquitoes are most active.
- Wear long-sleeved shirts and long pants when outdoors.
- Spray clothing or exposed skin with repellents containing DEET, following the manufacturer's guidelines. For children, the repellent should contain no more than 30% DEET. Use the smallest amount possible. It is necessary to repeat application of repellent approximately every 2 hours.

▶ Pertussis

Pertussis is caused by a bacterium and is a highly communicable respiratory infection. People of all ages may be affected, but it is most often diagnosed in children and infants. There is a characteristic paroxysmal "whooping" cough that is often followed by vomiting. Transmission occurs from person to person with direct contact to the infected secretions or mucous membranes of infected persons.

Symptoms

Symptoms include:
- Cough
- Shortness of breath
- Hypoxia (a condition in which the body's cells and tissues do not have enough oxygen)
- Pneumonia
- Seizures

Diagnosis

Diagnosis is made by clinical history, physical exam, and confirming laboratory tests.

Treatment

Pertussis is treated with antibiotics.

Prevention

Vaccination is available to prevent this disease. People exposed to an active case of pertussis are offered antibiotics to prevent the development of the disease.

> ## FYI
>
> **Pertussis**
> - Since 1990, there has been an increase in cases, disproportionately affecting adolescents and adults.
> - Before the availability of vaccine there were more than 200,000 cases of pertussis annually. Since then, there has been an average of 4,400 cases.
> - Recent evidence suggests that immunity from the disease may not be permanent.

▶ Rabies

Rabies is a virus that causes a fatal illness. Hosts for the virus include bats and carnivores, but the primary host for the virus varies from region to region. Most often transmitted from the bite of an infected animal, nonbite exposures do occur through open wounds and mucous membranes from contaminated areas such as caves.

Animals who change their behavior, show signs of problems swallowing or drooling, and display increased aggressive behaviors might be infected with the virus and should be avoided.

Symptoms

The symptoms are quite dramatic and include:
- Fever
- Headache
- Paralysis
- Spasms of swallowing muscles
- Spasms that may be triggered by the sight, sound, or perception of water
- Delirium
- Convulsions
- Coma

Diagnosis

Talk to your health care provider after being bitten by any animal. Decisions about use of rabies vaccination may be made by special studies performed on the brain tissue of the animal suspected of having rabies.

Treatment

If you are bitten by a potentially rabid animal, wash the wound with soap and water, and seek medical attention. Assessment of the risk for infection includes the geographic location where the bite incident occurred, the animal involved, and the vaccination status of that animal, if known. The use of postexposure immunization is indicated for persons who have been possibly exposed to a rabid animal. There have been no treatment failures within the United States when the vaccine is given promptly and appropriately.

Prevention

The primary means to control the rabies virus is to have pets vaccinated, to avoid handling wild animals, and to report to animal control personnel any animal acting strangely.

Pre-exposure vaccination is recommended for any person who must routinely handle animals or who might travel to areas around the world where his or her work may result in exposure to infected animals. Cavers or spelunkers should consider receiv-

FYI

Rabies

- Rabies is a virus that is found throughout the world on every continent except Antarctica.
- The word for rabies is derived from the Latin word that means "to rage."
- All mammals are believed to be susceptible to the virus.

ing pre-exposure vaccination, too. Bat droppings may be stirred into the air by movement through the cave, and dust from these droppings may contain rabies virus.

▶ Respiratory Syncytial Virus

Respiratory syncytial virus (RSV) is the most common cause of respiratory infections in children under 1 year of age. The disease is spread from close person-to-person contact. Infections most often occur from late fall to early spring.

Symptoms

Symptoms include:

- Fever
- Stuffy or runny nose
- Cough
- Wheezing

Diagnosis

Diagnosis is made by a combination of blood tests and tests of nasal secretions.

Treatment

No specific treatment is necessary, other than management of the symptoms. Most children will recover from the illness in 8 to 15 days. The majority of children hospitalized for RSV are under 6 months of age. RSV may cause severe disease in patients with compromised immune systems, heart disease, or other lung diseases.

Prevention

Wash hands frequently and do not share cups or glasses. Avoid contact with people who are coughing and sneezing.

▶ SARS

SARS first appeared in Southern China in November of 2002. It is a viral respiratory illness spread by close person-to-person contact, most likely through the respiratory droplets that result when a person coughs or sneezes. Close contact is defined as living with or caring for someone with SARS.

Symptoms

The symptoms are somewhat similar to the flu without sore throat and include:

- Fever (temperature over 100.4°F)
- Headache
- Body aches
- Cough that may develop 2 to 7 days after the onset of the illness
- Diarrhea in up to 20% of the patients
- Often severe pneumonia

Diagnosis

Risk of exposure and associated symptoms are taken into consideration. The likelihood that a person has SARS is very low unless the typical symptoms are present along with evidence of being at risk of exposure to the disease. Blood tests and other laboratory tests, as well as X-ray films, are used to confirm diagnosis.

Treatment

No specific treatment is currently available for SARS. If pneumonia develops, the Centers for Disease Control and Prevention (CDC) recommend that the person receive the same treatment as that used for any patient with a serious community-acquired, atypical pneumonia. Research is being performed to determine which antiviral medications are effective against this virus.

FYI

SARS
- Between November 2002 and July 2003, a total of 8,098 SARS cases were reported to the World Health Organization from 29 countries.
- In the United States, only eight people had laboratory evidence of infection with SARS.

Prevention

There is no specific prevention measure. Surveillance by governments and reporting of suspected cases by health care providers are critical for containing the spread of this virus. When traveling abroad, it is a good practice to check travel notices published by the CDC.

▶ *Shigella, Salmonella, E coli,* and *Giardia*

A variety of bacteria and parasites may cause watery or bloody diarrhea and abdominal cramps that are present with or without fever. Because the presentations of these illnesses are so similar, it is useful to consider them together.

Infection often arises as a result of a food-borne illness, such as eating undercooked meat, raw eggs, or drinking contaminated water or raw milk. Person-to-person contact is an especially important source of transmission in childcare facilities. Touching contaminated surfaces and wiping your nose or mouth may also cause infection.

Symptoms

Symptoms may include:
- Fever
- Frequent formed stools
- Watery, loose stools
- Bloody stools
- Abdominal cramps
- Foul odor to the stool
- Weight loss
- Dehydration

FYI

Shigella, Salmonella, E coli, and Giardia
- In the United States, about 18,000 people will become infected with *Shigella* each year. The disease is more common in the summer. Children who are 2 to 4 years of age are most likely to get the disease.
- *Salmonella* bacteria have become resistant to antibiotics as a result of the use of antibiotics by the agricultural industry to manage the growth of feed animals.
- *Salmonella typhi* is the bacterium that causes typhoid fever. *S typhi* lives only in humans and is carried in the bloodstream and intestines.
- *E coli* 0157:H7 is an emerging cause of serious illness, causing 73,000 cases of bloody diarrhea each year.
- *Giardia* is a one-celled organism. Found throughout the world, it is the most common cause of waterborne disease in humans.

Complications may arise with the invasion of the bacteria into the bloodstream. Symptoms may progress and include:
- Joint pain
- Painful urination
- Eye irritation
- Death

Diagnosis

In all cases, stool samples are requested, and samples will be sent for evaluation for both parasites and bacteria. The onset of illness is a valuable clue for determining the cause of diarrhea.

Treatment

Treatment will vary depending on the infection. Antibiotics are sometimes recommended. Antidiarrhea medications are usually avoided because they may delay clearing bacteria from the intestines. In many cases, the diarrhea resolves spontaneously.

Prevention

Wash hands frequently and thoroughly. Pay attention to how food is prepared. Drink water only from reliable areas or sources.

▶ Smallpox

Smallpox (Variola) is a virus that causes a serious and frequently fatal disease.

Symptoms

Symptoms include:
- Fever
- Malaise
- Body aches
- Headache
- Vomiting
- A rash that first appears in the mouth and on the tongue
- Firm, hard pustules on the skin
- Bleeding
- Shock
- Death

Diagnosis

Diagnosis is made by history and the appearance and progression of the rash. Diagnosis of any case of smallpox is a national emergency.

Treatment

Isolation is required, and treatment may be extensive, requiring fluid replacement, management of second-ary infections, nutritional support, airway management, and treatment of shock.

Prevention

Because smallpox no longer exists in the natural state, no prevention is necessary. Vaccination against the disease is part of a national strategy to respond to a terrorist threat. Because the vaccine does have some risk, only first responders have been offered the vaccine. Should an outbreak occur, vaccine would be offered to people at risk.

▶ Tularemia

Tularemia is a bacterium whose typical hosts are rodents and rabbits. Tularemia is found throughout the United States. Infection with tularemia is often called "rabbit fever." People become infected from a bite by an infected tick, deerfly, or other insect. Handling an infected animal or animal carcass may cause transmission of the disease.

Tularemia is highly infectious. It is not spread by person-to-person contact, and therefore, isolation of the infected person is not necessary.

Symptoms

Symptoms include:
- Sudden fever
- Chills
- Headache
- Diarrhea
- Muscle aches
- Joint pain
- Dry cough
- Weakness
- Pneumonia
- Death

FYI

Smallpox
- The last case of smallpox in the United States was in 1949. The last naturally occurring case in the entire world was in Somalia in 1977.
- The only source for infection with smallpox is from laboratory stockpiles.
- There is concern that these stockpiles might be stolen and used as a biological weapon by terrorists.

FYI

Tularemia
- Although the number of cases has substantially declined, tularemia outbreaks continue to occur across the United States.
- Tularemia is considered a potential biological weapon.

Route of exposure is associated with:

- Skin ulcers
- Painful lymph glands
- Swollen, painful eyes
- Sore throat

Diagnosis

Symptoms typically appear 2 to 5 days after exposure but may take up to 2 weeks to develop. Laboratory tests on blood and sputum may be used to diagnose the disease.

Treatment

Antibiotics are used to treat this disease. Treatment should begin as soon as possible. The disease may be fatal if not effectively treated.

Prevention

Because tularemia is naturally occurring in many parts of the United States, basic precautions are recommended, including using insect repellent containing DEET according to the manufacturer's instructions, washing hands often with soap and water or alcohol-based hand wash, and noting any change in pets or livestock and consulting with a veterinarian.

▶ Viral Hemorrhagic Fevers

The term *viral hemorrhagic fever* refers to a group of illnesses that may cause relatively mild diseases; however, some can cause serious life-threatening illness. The Ebola virus and the Marburg virus are the best known.

Ebola Hemorrhagic Fever

Ebola hemorrhagic fever was first recognized in the Democratic Republic of the Congo in 1976 and is named after the river in the region. The disease is severe, often fatal, and appears sporadically. The source of the virus remains unknown, but it is believed to have an animal host. Most cases have occurred around the Ebola river areas of Africa.

Infection with the Ebola virus is rapid with no carrier state. It is suspected that the first transmission is from an infected animal to a person. Thereafter,

people can become infected from exposure to a person who has the disease. Because it is spread from person to person through contact with blood or secretions, family members quickly become infected. Health care workers may become infected, and without adequate precautions, the disease may spread through a health care facility.

Symptoms

Incubation ranges from 2 to 21 days. The common symptoms include:

- Fever
- Headache
- Joint aches
- Muscle aches
- Sore throat

Other symptoms include:

- Diarrhea
- Vomiting
- Stomach pain
- Rash
- Red eyes
- Internal and external bleeding

FYI

Marburg Hemorrhagic Fever

- It was first recognized in 1967 from an outbreak that occurred in a laboratory in Marburg, Germany, where laboratory workers became ill while working with monkeys infected with the virus. The monkeys had been imported from Uganda. The infected workers subsequently spread the infection to family members and several of the medical staff treating them.
- The virus is rare, with reports of the illness occurring in 1976 and 1980.
- The actual animal source is unknown. After a person is infected, the disease spreads from person-to-person contact.
- The disease has a mortality rate of 30%, and recovery from the illness may take many weeks.

Diagnosis

The patient's history and the number of symptoms present are used to make the diagnosis. The rash and red eyes are not specific to the illness. There are specific blood tests to confirm the diagnosis.

Treatment

There is no standard treatment, but properly supporting the patient with medications, fluids, and oxygen is necessary.

Prevention

Prevention is difficult because often the source of the virus cannot be determined. Cases must be diagnosed rapidly to prevent spread, but diagnosis is often difficult because early symptoms are vague and nonspecific. Proper isolation techniques must be used, especially respiratory isolation. Unfortunately, oftentimes there have been multiple exposures before isolation has occurred. It is important to have a high index of suspicion for SARS to prevent its spread.

▶ Prevention Strategies

Respiratory Protections

Several varieties of masks and respirators are available for household and business use. Training in the proper use of the mask or respirator is often necessary as well as proper fit for the device to function properly. There are limitations to the effectiveness of masks and respirators. For example, facial hair does not permit the necessary seal, and the device will not work effectively. The decision to use a mask or respirator is not as important as the decision to avoid the exposure, if at all possible.

Effective protection requires:
- Correct mask or respirator for the specific hazard
- Correct fit for the device
- Availability when needed
- Device in proper working order
- Knowledge of proper methods for:
  - Donning
  - Wearing
  - Removing

Handwashing

Adherence to a consistent effort to wash hands with soap and water is the most sensible strategy to reduce risk for infection. When soap and water are not available, using an alcohol-based hand wash is strongly recommended. Hands should be washed frequently. It is a good habit to wash hands before consuming food and beverages.

Use common sense; if your hands are visibly dirty, then wash them! If you have gone into an area that is dirty, dusty, or might otherwise have contaminated surfaces, it is necessary to wash your hands as soon as possible after leaving the area. Carrying an alcohol-based hand wash with you will let you quickly cleanse your hands whenever necessary, but is not as effective as good handwashing. Effective handwashing requires a 10-second wash with soap, working up a lather over the entire hand, and rinsing well, preferably with warm water.

Site-Specific Work Page

Employee Training

Respiratory protection at the worksite: _____

The person at your facility who does fit testing is: _____

At my worksite, masks and respirators are available at the following locations: _____

Examples of times that I should consider using respiratory protection are:

A. _____

B. _____

C. _____

Limitations to the effectiveness of a respirator include:

A. _____

B. _____

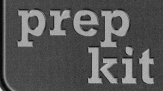

▶ Check Your Knowledge

1. Chicken pox and shingles are caused by the same virus.
   A. True
   B. False

2. Deer mouse urine and feces cause the spread of hantavirus.
   A. True
   B. False

3. Flu causes approximately 36,000 deaths each year in the United States.
   A. True
   B. False

4. West Nile virus was discovered in Cairo, Egypt.
   A. True
   B. False

5. DEET is not recommended for avoiding insect bites.
   A. True
   B. False

Answers: **1.** A; **2.** A; **3.** A; **4.** B; **5.** B

OSHA Bloodborne Pathogens Standard

Regulations Section 1910.1030

Part 1910-[Amended]
Subpart Z-[Amended]
1. The general authority citation for subpart Z of 29 CFR part 1910 continues to read as follows and a new citation for 1910.1030 is added:
Authority: Secs. 6 and 8, Occupational Safety and Health Act, 29 U.S.C. 655, 657, Secretary of Labor's Orders Nos. 12-71 (36 CFR 8754), 8-76 (41 CFR 25059), or 9-83 (48 CFR 35736), as applicable; and 29 CFR part 1911.

* * *

Section 1910.1030 also issued under 29 U.S.C. 853.

* * *

2. Section 1910.1030 is added to read as follows:
1910.1030 Bloodborne Pathogens.
(a) *Scope and Application*
This section applies to all occupational exposure to blood or other potentially infectious materials as defined by paragraph (b) of this section.
(b) *Definitions*
For purposes of this section, the following shall apply:

Assistant Secretary means the Assistant Secretary of Labor for Occupational Safety and Health, or designated representative.

Blood means human blood, human blood components, and products made from human blood.

Bloodborne Pathogens means pathogenic microorganisms that are present in human blood and can cause disease in humans. These pathogens include, but are not limited to, Hepatitis B Virus [HBV] and Human Immunodeficiency Virus [HIV].

Clinical Laboratory means a workplace where diagnostic or other screening procedures are performed on blood or other potentially infectious materials.

Contaminated means the presence or the reasonably anticipated presence of blood or other potentially infectious materials on an item or surface.

Contaminated Laundry means laundry which has been soiled with blood or other potentially infectious materials or may contain sharps.

Contaminated Sharps means any contaminated object that can penetrate the skin including, but not limited to, needles, scalpels, broken glass, broken capillary tubes, and exposed ends of dental wires.

Decontamination means the use of physical or chemical means to remove, inactivate, or destroy bloodborne pathogens on a surface or item to the point where they are no longer capable of transmitting infectious particles and the surface or item is rendered safe for handling, use, or disposal.

Director means the Director of the National Institute for Occupational Safety and Health, U.S. Department of Health and Human Services, or designated representative.

Engineering Controls means controls (e.g., sharps disposal containers, self-sheathing needles) that isolate or remove the bloodborne pathogens hazard from the workplace.

Exposure Incident means a specific eye, mouth, other mucous membrane, non-intact skin, or parenteral contact with blood or other potentially infectious materials that results from the performance of an employee's duties.

Handwashing Facilities means a facility providing an adequate supply of running potable water, soap, and single use towels or hot air drying machines.

Licensed Health Care Professional is a person whose legally permitted scope of practice allows him or her to independently perform the activities required by paragraph (f) Hepatitis B vaccination and Post-Exposure Evaluation and Follow-Up.

HBV means Hepatitis B Virus.

HIV means Human Immunodeficiency Virus.

Occupational Exposure means reasonably anticipated skin, eye, mucous membrane, or parenteral contact with blood or other potentially infectious materials that may result from the performance of an employee's duties.

Other Potentially Infectious Materials means:

(1) The following human body fluids: semen, vaginal secretions, cerebrospinal fluid, synovial fluid, pleural fluid, pericardial fluid, peritoneal fluid, amniotic fluid, saliva in dental procedures, any body fluid that is visibly contaminated with blood, and all body fluids in situations where it is difficult or impossible to differentiate between body fluids;

(2) Any unfixed tissue or organ (other than intact skin) from a human (living or dead); and

(3) HIV-containing cell or tissue cultures, organ cultures, and HIV- or HBV-containing culture medium or other solutions; and blood, organs, or other tissues from experimental animals infected with HIV or HBV.

Parenteral means piercing mucous membranes or the skin barrier through such events as needle sticks, human bites, cuts, and abrasions.

Personal Protective Equipment is specialized clothing or equipment worn by an employee for protection against a hazard. General work clothes (e.g., uniforms, pants, shirts, or blouses) not intended to function as protection against a hazard are not considered to be personal protective equipment.

Production Facility means a facility engaged in industrial-scale, large-volume, or high concentration production of HIV or HBV.

Regulated Waste means liquid or semi-liquid blood or other potentially infectious materials; contaminated items that would release blood or other potentially infectious materials in a liquid or semi-liquid state if compressed; items that are caked with dried blood or other potentially infectious materials and are capable of releasing these materials during handling; contaminated sharps; and pathological and microbiological wastes containing blood or other potentially infectious materials.

Research Laboratory means a laboratory producing or using research-laboratory-scale amounts of HIV or HBV. Research laboratories may produce high concentrations of HIV or HBV but not in the volume found in production facilities.

Source Individual means any individual, living or dead, whose blood or other potentially infectious materials may be a source of occupational exposure to the employee. Examples include, but are not limited to, hospital and clinic patients; clients in institutions for the developmentally disabled; trauma victims; clients of drug and alcohol treatment facilities; residents of hospices and nursing homes; human remains; and individuals who donate or sell blood or blood components.

Sterilize means the use of a physical or chemical procedure to destroy all microbial life including highly resistant bacterial endospores.

Universal Precautions is an approach to infection control. According to the concept of Universal Precautions, all human blood and certain human body fluids are treated as if known to be infectious for HIV, HBV, and other bloodborne pathogens.

Work Practice Controls means controls that reduce the likelihood of exposure by altering the manner in which a task is performed (e.g., prohibiting recapping of needles by a two-handed technique).

(c) **Exposure Control**

(1) *Exposure Control Plan.*

(i) Each employer having an employee(s) with occupational exposure as defined by paragraph (b) of this section shall establish a written Exposure Control Plan designed to eliminate or minimize employee exposure.

(ii) The Exposure Control Plan shall contain at least the following elements:

(A) The exposure determination required by paragraph (c)(2);

(B) The schedule and method of implementation for paragraphs (d) Methods of Compliance, (e) HIV and HBV Research Laboratories and Production Facilities, (f) Hepatitis B Vaccination and Post-Exposure Evaluation and Follow-Up,

(g) Communication of Hazards to Employees, and (h) Recordkeeping of this standard; and

(C) The procedure for the evaluation of circumstances surrounding exposure incidents as required by paragraph (f)(3)(i) of this standard.

(iii) Each employer shall ensure that a copy of the Exposure Control Plan is accessible to employees in accordance with 29 CFR 1910.20(e).

(iv) The Exposure Control Plan shall be reviewed and updated at least annually and whenever necessary to reflect new or modified tasks and procedures which affect occupational exposure and to reflect new or revised employee positions with occupational exposure.

(v) The Exposure Control Plan shall be made available to the Assistant Secretary and the Director upon request for examination and copying.

(2) *Exposure Determination.*

(i) Each employer who has an employee(s) with occupational exposure as defined by paragraph (b) of this section shall prepare an exposure determination. This exposure determination shall contain the following:

(A) A list of all job classifications in which all employees in those job classifications have occupational exposure;

(B) A list of job classifications in which some employees have occupational exposure; and

(C) A list of all tasks and procedures or groups of closely related task and procedures in which occupational exposures occur and that are performed by employees in job classifications listed in accordance with the provisions of paragraph (c)(2)(i)(B) of this standard.

(ii) This exposure determination shall be made without regard to the use of personal protective equipment.

(d) *Methods of Compliance*

(1) *General.*

Universal precautions shall be observed to prevent contact with blood or other potentially infectious materials. Under circumstances in which differentiation between body fluid types is difficult or impossible, all body fluids shall be considered potentially infectious materials.

(2) *Engineering and Work Practice Controls.*

(i) Engineering and work practice controls shall be used to eliminate or minimize employee exposure. Where occupational exposure remains after institution of these controls, personal protective equipment shall also be used.

(ii) Engineering controls shall be examined and maintained or replaced on a regular schedule to ensure their effectiveness.

(iii) Employers shall provide handwashing facilities which are readily accessible to employees.

(iv) When provision of handwashing facilities is not feasible, the employer shall provide either an appropriate antiseptic hand cleanser in conjunction with clean cloth/paper towels or antiseptic towelettes. When antiseptic hand cleansers or towelettes are used, hands shall be washed with soap and running water as soon as feasible.

(v) Employers shall ensure that employees wash their hands immediately or as soon as feasible after removal of gloves or other personal protective equipment.

(vi) Employers shall ensure that employees wash hands and any other skin with soap and water, or flush mucous membranes with water immediately or as soon as feasible following contact of such body areas with blood or other potentially infectious materials.

(vii) Contaminated needles and other contaminated sharps shall not be bent, recapped, or removed except as noted in paragraphs (d)(2)(vii)(A) and (d)(2)(vii)(B) below. Shearing or breaking of contaminated needles is prohibited.

(A) Contaminated needles and other contaminated sharps shall not be recapped or removed unless the employer can demonstrate that no alternative is feasible or that such action is required by a specific medical procedure.

(B) Such recapping or needle removal must be accomplished through the use of a mechanical device or a one-handed technique.

(viii) Immediately or as soon as possible after use, contaminated reusable sharps shall be placed in appropriate containers until properly reprocessed. These containers shall be:

(A) Puncture resistant;

(B) Labeled or color-coded in accordance with this standard;

(C) Leakproof on the sides and bottom; and

(D) In accordance with the requirements set forth in paragraph (d)(4)(ii)(E) for reusable sharps.

(ix) Eating, drinking, smoking, applying cosmetics or lip balm, and handling contact lenses are prohibited in work areas where there is a reasonable likelihood of occupational exposure.

(x) Food and drink shall not be kept in refrigerators, freezers, shelves, cabinets or on countertops or bench-tops where blood or other potentially infectious materials are present.

(xi) All procedures involving blood or other potentially infectious materials shall be performed in such a manner as to minimize splashing, spraying, spattering, and generation of droplets of these substances.

(xii) Mouth pipetting/suctioning of blood or other potentially infectious materials is prohibited.

(xiii) Specimens of blood or other potentially infectious materials shall be placed in a container which prevents leakage during collection, handling, processing, storage, transport, or shipping.

(A) The container for storage, transport, or shipping shall be labeled or color-coded according to paragraph (g)(1)(i) and closed prior to being stored, transported, or shipped. When a facility utilizes Universal Precautions in the handling of all specimens, the labeling/color-coding of specimens is not necessary provided containers are recognizable as containing specimens. This exemption only applies while such specimens/containers remain within the facility. Labeling or color-coding in accordance with paragraph (g)(1)(i) is required when such specimens/containers leave the facility.

(B) If outside contamination of the primary container occurs, the primary container shall be placed within a second container which prevents leakage during handling, processing, storage, transport, or shipping and is labeled or color-coded according to the requirements of this standard.

(C) If the specimen could puncture the primary container, the primary container shall be placed within a secondary container which is puncture-resistant in addition to the above characteristics.

(xiv) Equipment which may become contaminated with blood or other potentially infectious materials shall be examined prior to servicing or shipping and shall be decontaminated as necessary, unless the employer can demonstrate that decontamination of such equipment or portions of such equipment is not feasible.

(A) A readily observable label in accordance with paragraph

(g)(1)(i)(H) shall be attached to the equipment stating which portions remain contaminated.

(B) The employer shall ensure that this information is conveyed to all affected employees, the servicing representative, and/or the manufacturer, as appropriate, prior to handling, servicing, or shipping so that appropriate precautions will be taken.

(3) *Personal Protective Equipment.*

(i) Provision. When there is occupational exposure, the employer shall provide, at no cost to the employee, appropriate personal protective equipment such as, but not limited to, gloves, gowns, laboratory coats, face shields or masks and eye protection, and mouthpieces, resuscitation bags, pocket masks, or other ventilation devices. Personal protective equipment will be considered "appropriate" only if it does not permit blood or other potentially infectious materials to pass through to or reach the employee's work clothes, street clothes, undergarments, skin, eyes, mouth, or other mucous membranes under normal conditions of use and for the duration of time which the protective equipment will be used.

(ii) Use. The employer shall ensure that the employee uses appropriate personal protective equipment unless the employer shows that the employee temporarily and briefly declined to use personal protective equipment when, under rare and extraordinary circumstances, it was the employee's professional judgment that in the specific instance its use would have prevented the delivery of health care or public safety services or would have posed an increased hazard to the safety of the worker or co-worker. When the employee makes this judgment, the circumstances shall be investigated and documented in order to determine whether changes can be instituted to prevent such occurrences in the future.

(iii) Accessibility. The employer shall ensure that appropriate personal protective equipment in the appropriate sizes is readily accessible at the worksite or is issued to employees. Hypoallergenic gloves, glove liners, powderless gloves, or other similar alternatives shall be readily accessible to those employees who are allergic to the gloves normally provided.

(iv) Cleaning, Laundering, and Disposal. The employer shall clean, launder, and dispose of personal protective equipment required by paragraphs (d) and (e) of this standard, at no cost to the employee.

(v) Repair and Replacement. The employer shall repair or replace personal protective equipment as needed to maintain its effectiveness, at no cost to the employee.

(vi) If a garment(s) is penetrated by blood or other potentially infectious materials, the garment(s) shall be removed immediately or as soon as feasible.

(vii) All personal protective equipment shall be removed prior to leaving the work area.

(viii) When personal protective equipment is removed it shall be placed in an appropriately designated area or container for storage, washing, decontamination, or disposal.

(ix) Gloves. Gloves shall be worn when it can be reasonably anticipated that the employee may have hand contact with blood, other potentially infectious materials, mucous membranes, and non-intact skin; when performing vascular access procedures except as specified in paragraph (d)(3)(ix)(D); and when handling or touching contaminated items or surfaces.

(A) Disposable (single-use) gloves such as surgical or examination gloves, shall be replaced as soon as practical when contaminated or as soon as feasible if they are torn, punctured, or when their ability to function as a barrier is compromised.

(B) Disposable (single-use) gloves shall not be washed or decontaminated for re-use.

(C) Utility gloves may be decontaminated for reuse if the integrity of the glove is not compromised. However, they must be discarded if they are cracked, peeling, torn, punctured, or exhibit other signs of deterioration or when their ability to function as a barrier is compromised.

(D) If an employer in a volunteer blood donation center judges that routine gloving for all phlebotomies is not necessary then the employer shall:

  (1) Periodically reevaluate this policy;

  (2) Make gloves available to all employees who wish to use them for phlebotomy;

  (3) Not discourage the use of gloves for phlebotomy; and

  (4) Require that gloves be used for phlebotomy in the following circumstances:

  (i) When the employee has cuts, scratches, or other breaks in his or her skin;

  (ii) When the employee judges that hand contamination with blood may occur, for example, when performing phlebotomy on an uncooperative source individual; and

  (iii) When the employee is receiving training in phlebotomy.

(x) Masks, Eye Protection, and Face Shields. Masks in combination with eye protection devices, such as goggles or glasses with solid side shields, or chin-length face shields, shall be worn whenever splashes, spray, spatter, or droplets of blood or other potentially infectious materials may be generated and eye, nose, or mouth contamination can be reasonably anticipated.

(xi) Gowns, Aprons, and Other Protective Body Clothing. Appropriate protective clothing such as, but not limited to, gowns, aprons, lab coats, clinic jackets, or similar outer garments shall be worn in occupational exposure situations. The type and characteristics will depend upon the task and degree of exposure anticipated.

(xii) Surgical caps or hoods and/or shoe covers or boots shall be worn in instances when gross contamination can reasonably be anticipated (e.g., autopsies, orthopedic surgery).

(4) *Housekeeping.*

  (i) General. Employers shall ensure that the worksite is maintained in a clean and sanitary condition. The employer shall determine and implement an appropriate written schedule for cleaning and method of decontamination based upon the location within the facility, type of surface to be cleaned, type of soil present, and tasks or procedures being performed in the area.

  (ii) All equipment and environmental and working surfaces shall be cleaned and decontaminated after contact with blood or other potentially infectious materials.

  (A) Contaminated work surfaces shall be decontaminated with an appropriate disinfectant after completion of procedures; immediately or as soon as feasible when surfaces are overtly contaminated or after any spill of blood or other potentially infectious materials; and at the end of the work shift if the surface may have become contaminated since the last cleaning.

(B) Protective coverings, such as plastic wrap, aluminum foil, or imperviously backed absorbent paper used to cover equipment and environmental surfaces, shall be removed and replaced as soon as feasible when they become overtly contaminated or at the end of the work shift if they may have become contaminated during the shift.

(C) All bins, pails, cans, and similar receptacles intended for reuse which have a reasonable likelihood for becoming contaminated with blood or other potentially infectious materials shall be inspected and decontaminated on a regularly scheduled basis and cleaned and decontaminated immediately or as soon as feasible upon visible contamination.

(D) Broken glassware which may be contaminated shall not be picked up directly with the hands. It shall be cleaned up using mechanical means, such as a brush and dust pan, tongs, or forceps.

(E) Reusable sharps that are contaminated with blood or other potentially infectious materials shall not be stored or processed in a manner that requires employees to reach by hand into the containers where these sharps have been placed.

(iii) Regulated Waste.

  (A) Contaminated Sharps Discarding and Containment.

    (1) Contaminated sharps shall be discarded immediately or as soon as feasible in containers that are:

    (i) Closable;

    (ii) Puncture resistant;

    (iii) Leakproof on sides and bottom; and

    (iv) Labeled or color-coded in accordance with paragraph (g)(1)(i) of this standard.

(2) During use, containers for contaminated sharps shall be:

(i) Easily accessible to personnel and located as close as is feasible to the immediate area where sharps are used or can be reasonably anticipated to be found (e.g., laundries);

(ii) Maintained upright throughout use; and

(iii) Replaced routinely and not be allowed to overfill.

(3) moving containers of contaminated sharps from the area of use, the containers shall be:

(i) Closed immediately prior to removal or replacement to prevent spillage or protrusion of contents during handling, storage, transport, or shipping;

(ii) Placed in a secondary container if leakage is possible. The second container shall be:

(A) Closable;

(B) Constructed to contain all contents and prevent leakage during handling, storage, transport, or shipping; and

(C) Labeled or color-coded according to paragraph (g)(1)(i) of this standard.

(4) Reusable containers shall not be opened, emptied, or cleaned manually or in any other manner which would expose employees to the risk of percutaneous injury.

(B) Regulated Waste Containment.

  (1) Regulated waste shall be placed in containers that are:

  (i) Closable;

  (ii) Constructed to contain all contents and prevent leakage of fluids during handling, storage, transport, or shipping;

  (iii) Labeled or color-coded in accordance with paragraph (g)(1)(i) of this standard; and

(iv) Closed prior to removal to prevent spillage or protrusion of contents during handling, storage, transport, or shipping.

(2) If outside contamination of the regulated waste container occurs, it shall be placed in a second container. The second container shall be:

(i) Closable;

(ii) Constructed to contain all contents and prevent leakage of fluids during handling, storage, transport, or shipping;

(iii) Labeled or color-coded in accordance with paragraph (g)(1)(i) of this standard; and

(iv) Closed prior to removal to prevent spillage or protrusion of contents during handling, storage, transport, or shipping.

(C) Disposal of all regulated waste shall be in accordance with applicable regulations of the United States, States and Territories, and political subdivisions of States and Territories.

(iv) Laundry.

(A) Contaminated laundry shall be handled as little as possible with a minimum of agitation.

(1) Contaminated laundry shall be bagged or containerized at the location where it was used and shall not be sorted or rinsed in the location of use.

(2) Contaminated laundry shall be placed and transported in bags or containers labeled or color-coded in accordance with paragraph (g)(1)(i) of this standard. When a facility utilizes Universal Precautions in the handling of all soiled laundry, alternative labeling or color-coding is sufficient if it permits all employees to recognize the containers as requiring compliance with Universal Precautions.

(3) Whenever contaminated laundry is wet and presents a reasonable likelihood of soak-through of or leakage from the bag or container, the laundry shall be placed and transported in bags or containers which prevent soak-through and/or leakage of fluids to the exterior.

(B) The employer shall ensure that employees who have contact with contaminated laundry wear protective gloves and other appropriate personal protective equipment.

(C) When a facility ships contaminated laundry off-site to a second facility which does not utilize Universal Precautions in the handling of all laundry, the facility generating the contaminated laundry must place such laundry in bags or containers which are labeled or color-coded in accordance with paragraph (g)(1)(i).

(e) **HIV and HBV Research Laboratories and Production Facilities.**

(1) This paragraph applies to research laboratories and production facilities engaged in the culture, production, concentration, experimentation, and manipulation of HIV and HBV. It does not apply to clinical or diagnostic laboratories engaged solely in the analysis of blood, tissues, or organs. These requirements apply in addition to the other requirements of the standard.

(2) Research laboratories and production facilities shall meet the following criteria:

(i) Standard microbiological practices. All regulated waste shall either be incinerated or decontaminated by a method such as autoclaving known to effectively destroy bloodborne pathogens.

(ii) Special practices:

(A) Laboratory doors shall be kept closed when work involving HIV or HBV is in progress.

(B) Contaminated materials that are to be decontaminated at a site away from the work area shall be placed in a durable, leakproof, labeled or color-coded container that is closed before being removed from the work area.

(C) Access to the work area shall be limited to authorized persons. Written policies and procedures shall be established whereby only persons who have been advised of the potential biohazard, who meet any specific entry requirements, and who comply with all entry and exit procedures shall be allowed to enter the work areas and animal rooms.

(D) When other potentially infectious materials or infected animals are present in the work area or containment module, a hazard warning sign incorporating the universal biohazard symbol shall be posted on all access doors. The hazard warning sign shall comply with paragraph (g)(1)(ii) of this standard.

(E) All activities involving other potentially infectious materials shall be conducted in biological safety cabinets or other physical-containment devices within the containment module. No work with these other potentially infectious materials shall be conducted on the open bench.

(F) Laboratory coats, gowns, smocks, uniforms, or other appropriate protective clothing shall be used in the work area and animal rooms. Protective clothing shall not be worn outside of the work area and shall be decontaminated before being laundered.

(G) Special care shall be taken to avoid skin contact with other potentially infectious materials. Gloves shall be worn when handling infected animals and when making hand contact with other potentially infectious materials is unavoidable.

(H) Before disposal all waste from work areas and from animal rooms shall either be incinerated or decontaminated by a method such as autoclaving known to effectively destroy bloodborne pathogens.

(I) Vacuum lines shall be protected with liquid disinfectant traps and high efficiency particulate air (HEPA) filters or filters of equivalent or superior efficiency and which are checked routinely and maintained or replaced as necessary.

(J) Hypodermic needles and syringes shall be used only for parenteral injection and aspiration of fluids from laboratory animals and diaphragm bottles. Only needle-locking syringes or disposable syringe-needle units (i.e., the needle is integral to the syringe) shall be used for the injection or aspiration of other potentially infectious materials. Extreme caution shall be used when handling needles and syringes. A needle shall not be bent, sheared, replaced in the sheath or guard, or removed from the syringe following use. The needle and syringe shall be promptly placed in a puncture-resistant container and autoclaved or decontaminated before reuse or disposal.

(K) All spills shall be immediately contained and cleaned up by appropriate professional staff or others properly trained and equipped to work with potentially concentrated infectious materials.

(L) A spill or accident that results in an exposure incident shall be immediately reported to the laboratory director or other responsible person.

(M) A biosafety manual shall be prepared or adopted and periodically reviewed and updated at least annually or more often if necessary. Personnel shall be advised of potential hazards, shall be required to read instructions on practices and procedures, and shall be required to follow them.

(iii) Containment Equipment.

    (A) Certified biological safety cabinets (Class II, III, or IV) or other appropriate combinations of personal protection or physical containment devices, such as special protective clothing, respirators, centrifuge safety cups, sealed centrifuge rotors, and containment caging for animals, shall be used for all activities with other potentially infectious materials that pose a threat of exposure to droplets, splashes, spills, or aerosols.

    (B) Biological safety cabinets shall be certified when installed, whenever they are moved, and at least annually.

(3) HIV and HBV research laboratories shall meet the following criteria:

    (i) Each laboratory shall contain a facility for handwashing and an eye wash facility which is readily available within the work area.

    (ii) An autoclave for decontamination or regulated waste shall be available.

(4) HIV and HBV production facilities shall meet the following criteria:

    (i) The work areas shall be separated from areas that are open to unrestricted traffic flow within the building. Passage through two sets of doors shall be the basic requirement for entry into the work area from access corridors or other contiguous areas. Physical separation of the high-containment work area from access corridors or other areas or activities may also be provided by a double-doored clothes-change room (showers may be included), airlock, or other access facility that requires passing through two sets of doors before entering the work area.

    (ii) The surfaces of doors, walls, floors, and ceilings in the work area shall be water resistant so that they can be easily cleaned. Penetrations in these surfaces shall be sealed or capable of being sealed to facilitate decontamination.

    (iii) Each work area shall contain a sink for washing hands and readily available eye wash facility. The sink shall be foot, elbow, or automatically operated and shall be located near the exit door of the work area.

    (iv) Access doors to the work area or containment module shall be self-closing.

    (v) An autoclave for decontamination of regulated waste shall be available within or as near as possible to the work area.

    (vi) A ducted exhaust-air ventilation system shall be provided. This system shall create directional airflow that draws air into the work area through the entry area. The exhaust air shall not be recirculated to any other area of the building, shall be discharged to the outside, and shall be dispersed away from occupied areas and air intakes. The proper direction of the airflow shall be verified (i.e., into the work area).

(5) *Training Requirements.*

Additional training requirements for employees in HIV and HBV research laboratories and HIV and HBV production facilities are specified in paragraph (g)(2)(ix).

(f) *Hepatitis B Vaccination and Post-Exposure Evaluation and Follow-Up.*

(1) *General.*

    (i) The employer shall make available the Hepatitis B vaccine and vaccination series to all employees who have occupational exposure, and post-exposure evaluation and follow-up to all employees who have had an exposure incident.

(ii) The employer shall ensure that all medical evaluations and procedures including the Hepatitis B vaccine and vaccination series and post-exposure evaluation and follow-up, including prophylaxis, are:

  (A) Made available at no cost to the employee;

  (B) Made available to the employee at a reasonable time and place;

  (C) Performed by or under the supervision of a licensed physician or by or under the supervision of another licensed health care professional; and

  (D) Provided according to recommendations of the U.S. Public Health Service current at the time these evaluations and procedures take place, except as specified by this paragraph (f).

(iii) The employer shall ensure that all laboratory tests are conducted by an accredited laboratory at no cost to the employee.

(2) *Hepatitis B Vaccination.*

(i) Hepatitis B vaccination shall be made available after the employee has received the training required in paragraph (g)(2)(vii)(I) and within 10 working days of initial assignment to all employees who have occupational exposure unless the employee has previously received the complete Hepatitis B vaccination series, antibody testing has revealed that the employee is immune, or the vaccine is contraindicated for medical reasons.

(ii) The employer shall not make participation in a prescreening program a prerequisite for receiving Hepatitis B vaccination.

(iii) If the employee initially declines Hepatitis B vaccination but at a later date while still covered under the standard decides to accept the vaccination, the employer shall make available Hepatitis B vaccination at that time.

(iv) The employer shall assure that employees who decline to accept Hepatitis B vaccination offered by the employer sign the statement in Appendix A.

(v) If a routine booster dose(s) of Hepatitis B vaccine is recommended by the U.S. Public Health Service at a future date, such booster dose(s) shall be made available in accordance with section (f)(1)(ii).

(3) *Post-Exposure Evaluation and Follow-Up.* Following a report of an exposure incident, the employer shall make immediately available to the exposed employee a confidential medical evaluation and follow-up, including at least the following elements:

(i) Documentation of the route(s) of exposure, and the circumstances under which the exposure incident occurred;

(ii) Identification and documentation of the source individual, unless the employer can establish that identification is infeasible or prohibited by state or local law:

  (A) The source individual's blood shall be tested as soon as feasible and after consent is obtained in order to determine HBV and HIV infectivity. If consent is not obtained, the employer shall establish that legally required consent cannot be obtained. When the source individual's consent is not required by law, the source individual's blood, if available, shall be tested and the results documented.

  (B) When the source individual is already known to be infected with HBV or HIV, testing for the source individual's known HBV or HIV status need not be repeated.

(C) Results of the source individual's testing shall be made available to the exposed employee, and the employee shall be informed of applicable laws and regulations concerning disclosure of the identity and infectious status of the source individual.

(iii) Collection and testing of blood for HBV and HIV serological status:

(A) The exposed employee's blood shall be collected as soon as feasible and tested after consent is obtained.

(B) If the employee consents to baseline blood collection, but does not give consent at that time for HIV serologic testing, the sample shall be preserved for at least 90 days. If, within 90 days of the exposure incident, the employee elects to have the baseline sample tested, such testing shall be done as soon as feasible.

(iv) Post-exposure prophylaxis, when medically indicated, as recommended by the U.S. Public Health Service;

(v) Counseling; and

(vi) Evaluation of reported illnesses.

(4) *Information Provided to the Health Care Professional.*

(i) The employer shall ensure that the health care professional responsible for the employee's Hepatitis B vaccination is provided a copy of this regulation.

(ii) The employer shall ensure that the health care professional evaluating an employee after an exposure incident is provided the following information:

(A) A copy of this regulation;

(B) A description of the exposed employee's duties as they relate to the exposure incident;

(C) Documentation of the route(s) of exposure and circumstances under which the exposure occurred;

(D) Results of the source individual's blood testing, if available; and

(E) All medical records relevant to the appropriate treatment of the employee including vaccination status which are the employer's responsibility to maintain.

(5) *Health Care Professional's Written Opinion.* The employer shall obtain and provide the employee with a copy of the evaluating health care professional's written opinion within 15 days of the completion of the evaluation.

(i) The health care professional's written opinion for Hepatitis B vaccination shall be limited to whether Hepatitis B vaccination is indicated for an employee, and if the employee has received such vaccination.

(ii) The health care professional's written opinion for post-exposure evaluation and follow-up shall be limited to the following information:

(A) That the employee has been informed of the results of the evaluation; and

(B) That the employee has been told about any medical conditions resulting from exposure to blood or other potentially infectious materials which require further evaluation or treatment.

(iii) All other findings or diagnoses shall remain confidential and shall not be included in the written report.

(6) *Medical Recordkeeping.* Medical records required by this standard shall be maintained in accordance with paragraph (h)(1) of this section.

(g) *Communication of Hazards to Employees.*

(1) *Labels and Signs*

(i) Labels

(A) Warning labels shall be affixed to containers of regulated waste, refrigerators and freezers containing blood or other potentially infectious material; and other containers used to store, transport, or ship blood or other potentially infectious materials, except as provided in paragraph (g)(1)(i)(E), (F), and (G).

(B) Labels required by this section shall include the BIOHAZARD legend:

BIOHAZARD

(C) These labels shall be fluorescent orange or orange-red or predominantly so, with lettering or symbols in contrasting color.

(D) Labels shall be affixed as close as feasible to the container by string, wire, adhesive, or other method that prevents their loss or unintentional removal.

(E) Red bags or red containers may be substituted for labels.

(F) Containers of blood, blood components, or blood products that are labeled as to their contents and have been released for transfusion or other clinical use are exempted from labeling requirements of paragraph (g).

(G) Individual containers of blood or other potentially infectious materials that are placed in a labeled container during storage, transport, shipment, or disposal are exempted from the labeling requirement.

(H) Labels required for contaminated equipment shall be in accordance with this paragraph and shall also state which portions of the equipment remain contaminated.

(I) Regulated waste that has been decontaminated need not be labeled or color-coded.

(ii) Signs.

(A) The employer shall post signs at the entrance to work areas specified in paragraph (e), HIV and HBV Research Laboratory and Production Facilities, which shall bear the [BIOHAZARD] legend.

BIOHAZARD
(Name of the Infectious Agent) (Special requirements for entering the area) (Name, telephone number of the laboratory director or other responsible person)

(B) These signs shall be fluorescent orange-red or predominantly so, with lettering or symbols in a contrasting color.

(2) *Information and Training.*

(i) Employers shall ensure that all employees with occupational exposure participate in a training program which must be provided at no cost to the employee and during working hours.

(ii) Training shall be provided as follows:

(A) At the time of initial assignment to tasks where occupational exposure may take place;

(B) Within 90 days after the effective date of the standard; and

(C) At least annually thereafter.

(iii) For employees who have received training on bloodborne pathogens in the year preceding the effective date of the standard, only training with respect to the provisions of the standard which were not included need be provided.

(iv) Annual training for all employees shall be provided within one year of their previous training.

(v) Employers shall provide additional training when changes such as modification of tasks or procedures or institution of new tasks or procedures affect the employee's occupational exposure. The additional training may be limited to addressing the new exposures created.

(vi) Material appropriate in content and vocabulary to educational level, literacy, and language of employees shall be used.

(vii) The training program shall contain at a minimum the following elements:

(A) An accessible copy of the regulatory text of this standard and an explanation of its contents;

(B) A general explanation of the epidemiology and symptoms of bloodborne diseases;

(C) An explanation of the modes of transmission of bloodborne pathogens;

(D) An explanation of the employer's exposure control plan and the means by which the employee can obtain a copy of the written plan;

(E) An explanation of the appropriate methods for recognizing tasks and other activities that may involve exposure to blood and other potentially infectious materials;

(F) An explanation of the use and limitations of methods that will prevent or reduce exposure including appropriate engineering controls, work practices, and personal protective equipment;

(G) Information on the types, proper use, location, removal, handling, decontamination, and disposal of personal protective equipment;

(H) An explanation of the basis for selection of personal protective equipment;

(I) Information on the Hepatitis B vaccine, including information on its efficacy, safety, method of administration, the benefits of being vaccinated, and that the vaccine and vaccination will be offered free of charge;

(J) Information on the appropriate actions to take and persons to contact in an emergency involving blood or other potentially infectious materials;

(K) An explanation of the procedure to follow if an exposure incident occurs, including the method of reporting the incident and the medical follow-up that will be made available;

(L) Information on the post-exposure evaluation and follow-up that the employer is required to provide for the employee following an exposure incident;

(M) An explanation of the signs and labels and/or color-coding required by paragraph (g)(1); and

(N) An opportunity for interactive questions and answers with the person conducting the training session.

(viii) The person conducting the training shall be knowledgeable in the subject matter covered by the elements contained in the training program as it relates to the workplace that the training will address.

(ix) Additional Initial Training for Employees in HIV and HBV Laboratories and Production Facilities. Employees in HIV or HBV research laboratories and HIV or HBV production facilities shall receive the following initial training in addition to the above training requirements:

(A) The employer shall assure that employees demonstrate proficiency in standard micro-biological practices and techniques and in the practices and operations specific to the facility before being allowed to work with HIV or HBV.

(B) The employer shall assure that employees have prior experience in the handling of human pathogens or tissue cultures before working with HIV or HBV.

(C) The employer shall provide a training program to employees who have no prior experience in handling human pathogens. Initial work activities shall not include the handling of infectious agents. A progression of work activities shall be assigned as techniques are learned and proficiency is developed. The employer shall assure that employees participate in work activities involving infectious agents only after proficiency has been demonstrated.

(h) *Recordkeeping.*

   (1) *Medical Records*

   (i) The employer shall establish and maintain an accurate record for each employee with occupational exposure, in accordance with 29 CFR 1910.20.

   (ii) This record shall include:

   (A) The name and social security number of the employee;

   (B) A copy of the employee's Hepatitis B vaccination status including the dates of all the Hepatitis B vaccinations and any medical records relative to the employee's ability to receive vaccination as required by paragraph (f)(2);

   (C) A copy of all results of examinations, medical testing, and follow-up procedures as required by paragraph (f)(3);

   (D) The employer's copy of the health care professional's written opinion as required by paragraph (f)(5); and

   (E) A copy of the information provided to the health care professional as required by paragraphs (f)(4)(ii)(B), (C), and (D).

   (iii) Confidentiality. The employer shall ensure that employee medical records required by paragraph (h)(1) are:

   (A) Kept confidential; and

   (B) Not disclosed or reported without the employee's express written consent to any person within or outside the workplace except as required by this section or as may be required by law.

   (iv) The employer shall maintain the records required by paragraph (h) for at least the duration of employment plus 30 years in accordance with 29 CFR 1910.20.

   (2) *Training Records*

   (i) Training records shall include the following information:

   (A) The dates of the training sessions;

   (B) The contents or a summary of the training sessions;

   (C) The names and qualifications for the persons conducting the training; and

   (D) The names and job titles of all persons attending the training sessions.

   (ii) Training records shall be maintained for 3 years from the date on which the training occurred.

   (3) *Availability*

   (i) The employer shall ensure that all records required to be maintained by this section shall be made available upon request to the Assistant Secretary and Director for examination and copying.

   (ii) Employee training records required by this paragraph shall be provided upon request for examination and copying to employees, to employee representatives, to the Director, and to the Assistant Secretary in accordance with 29 CFR 1910.20.

   (iii) Employee medical records required by this paragraph shall be provided upon request for examination and copying to the subject employee, to anyone having written consent of the subject employee, to the Director, and to the Assistant Secretary in accordance with 29 CFR 1910.20

   (4) *Transfer of Records*

   (i) The employer shall comply with the requirements involving transfer of records set forth in 29 CFR 1910.20(h).

   (ii) If the employer ceases to do business and there is no successor employer to receive and retain the records for the prescribed period, the employer shall notify the Director, at least three months prior to their disposal and transmit them to the Director, if required by the Director to do so, within that three month period.

(i) Dates.

(1) Effective Date. The standard shall become effective on March 6, 1992.

(2) The Exposure Control Plan required by paragraph (c)(1) of this section shall be completed on or before May 5, 1992.

(3) Paragraph (g)(2) Information and Training and (h) Recordkeeping shall take effect on or before June 4, 1992.

(4) Paragraphs (d)(2) Engineering and Work Practice Controls, (d)(3) Personal Protective Equipment, (d)(4), Housekeeping, (e) HIV and HBV Research Laboratories and Production Facilities, (f) Hepatitis B Vaccination and Post-Exposure Evaluation and Follow-Up, and (g)(1) Labels and Signs shall take effect July 6, 1992.

Appendix A to Section 1910.1030—

Hepatitis B Vaccine Declination (Mandatory)

I understand that because of my occupational exposure to blood or other potentially infectious materials I may be at risk of acquiring hepatitis B virus (HBV) infection. I have been given the opportunity to be vaccinated with hepatitis B vaccine, at no charge to myself; however, I decline the hepatitis B vaccination at this time. I understand that by declining this vaccine, I continue to be at risk of acquiring hepatitis B, a serious disease. If in the future, I continue to have occupational exposure to blood or other potentially infectious materials, and I want to be vaccinated with hepatitis B vaccine. I can receive the vaccination series at no charge to me.

Appendix B

Hepatitis B Vaccine Declination Form

Appendix A to Section 1910.1030–Hepatitis B Vaccine Declination (Mandatory)

I understand that because of my occupational exposure to blood or other potentially infectious materials I may be at risk of acquiring hepatitis B virus (HBV) infection. I have been given the opportunity to be vaccinated with hepatitis B vaccine, at no charge to myself; however, I decline the hepatitis B vaccination at this time. I understand that by declining this vaccine, I continue to be at risk of acquiring hepatitis B, a serious disease. If in the future, I continue to have occupational exposure to blood or other potentially infectious materials, and I want to be vaccinated with hepatitis B vaccine. I can receive the vaccination series at no charge to me.

Employee Signature: _____

Date: _____

Employer Signature: _____

Date: _____

Sample Exposure Control Plan

This sample plan is provided as a guide to assist in complying with 29 CFR 1910.1030, OSHA's Bloodborne Pathogens Standard. It is not intended to supersede the requirements detailed in the standard. Employers should review the standard for particular requirements that are applicable to their specific situation. It should be noted that this model program does not include provisions for HIV/ HBV laboratories and research facilities that are addressed in section (e) of the standard. Employers operating these laboratories need to include provisions as required by the standard. Employers will need to add information relevant to their particular facility in order to develop an effective, comprehensive exposure control plan. Employers should note that the exposure control plan is expected to be reviewed at least on an annual basis and updated when necessary.

Bloodborne Pathogens Exposure Control Plan

Facility Name: _____

Date of Preparation: _____

Program Administration

(**Name of responsible person or department**) is (are) responsible for the implementation of the ECP. (**Name of responsible person or department**) will maintain, review, and update the ECP at least annually and whenever necessary to include new or modified tasks and procedures. Contact location/phone number: Those employees who are determined to have occupational exposure to blood or other potentially infectious materials (OPIMs) must comply with the procedures and work practices outlined in this ECP.

(**Name of responsible person or department**) will maintain and provide all necessary personal protective equipment (PPE), engineering controls (e.g., sharps containers), labels, and red bags as required by the standard. (**Name of responsible person or de-partment**) will ensure that adequate supplies of the aforementioned equipment are available in the appropriate sizes. Contact location/ phone number: _____.

(**Name of responsible person or department**) will be responsible for ensuring that all medical actions required are performed and that appropriate employee health and OSHA records are maintained. Contact location/phone number: _____.

(**Name of responsible person or department**) will be responsible for training, documentation of training, and making the written ECP available to employees, OSHA, and NIOSH representatives. Contact location/phone number: _____.

Exposure Control Plan

Employees covered by the bloodborne pathogens standard receive an explanation of this ECP during their initial training session. It will also be reviewed in their annual refresher training. All employees have an opportunity to review this plan at any time during their work shifts by contacting (**Name of responsible person or department**). If requested, we will provide an employee with a copy of the ECP free of charge and within 15 days of the request.

(**Name of responsible person or department**) is responsible for reviewing and updating the ECP annually or more frequently if necessary to reflect any new or modified tasks and procedures that affect occupational exposure and to reflect new or revised employee positions with occupational exposure.

In accordance with the OSHA Bloodborne Pathogens Standard, 29 CFR 1910.1030, the following exposure control plan has been developed.

1. Exposure Determination

OSHA requires employers to perform an exposure determination concerning which employees may incur occupational exposure to blood or other potentially infectious materials. The exposure determination is made without regard to the use of personal protective equipment (i.e., employees are considered to be exposed even if they wear personal protective equipment). This exposure determination is required to list all job classifications in which all employees may be expected to incur such occupational exposure, regardless of frequency. At this facility the following job classifications are in this category: _____.

In addition, OSHA requires a listing of job classifications in which some employees may have occupational exposure. Because not all the employees in these categories would be expected to incur exposure to blood or OPIMs, tasks or procedures that would cause these employees to have occupational exposure must also be listed in order to understand clearly which employees in these categories are considered to have occupational exposure. The job classifications and associated tasks for these categories are as follows:

Job Classification	Tasks/Procedures
_____	_____
_____	_____
_____	_____

2. Implementation Schedule and Method

OSHA also requires that this plan include a schedule and method of implementation for the various requirements of the standard.

Compliance Methods

Universal precautions will be observed at this facility in order to prevent contact with blood or other potentially infectious materials. All blood or other potentially infectious material will be considered infectious regardless of the perceived status of the source individual.

Engineering and work practice controls will be used to eliminate or minimize exposure to employees at this facility. Where occupational exposure remains after institution of these controls, personal protective equipment shall also be used. At this facility, the following engineering controls will be used: _____ (list controls, such as sharps containers).

These controls will be examined and maintained on a regular schedule. The schedule for reviewing the effectiveness of the controls is as follows: _____ (list schedule, such as daily or once/week, as well as who is responsible for reviewing the effectiveness of the individual controls, such as the supervisor for each department).

Handwashing facilities are also available to the employees who incur exposure to blood or other potentially infectious materials. OSHA requires that these facilities be readily accessible after incurring exposure. At this facility, handwashing facilities are located: (list locations, such as patient rooms, procedure area, etc.). If handwashing facilities are not feasible, the employer is required to provide either an antiseptic cleanser in conjunction with a clean cloth/paper towels or antiseptic towelettes. If these alternatives are used, then the hands are to be washed with soap and running water as soon as feasible.

Employers who must provide an alternative to readily accessible handwashing facilities should list the location, tasks, and responsibilities to ensure maintenance and accessibility of these alternatives.

After removal of personal protective gloves, employees shall wash hands and any other potentially contaminated skin area immediately or as soon as feasible with soap and water.

If employees incur exposure to their skin or mucous membranes, then those areas shall be washed or flushed with water as appropriate as soon as feasible after contact.

Needles

Contaminated needles and other contaminated sharps will not be bent, recapped, removed, sheared, or purposely broken. OSHA allows an exception to this if the procedure would require that the contaminated needles be recapped or removed and no alternative is feasible and the action is required by the medical procedure. If such action is required, then the recapping or removal of the needle must be done by the use of a mechanical device or a one-handed technique. At this facility, recapping or removal is only permitted for the following procedures: _____ (list the procedures and also list either the mechanical device to be used or alternatively if a one-handed technique will be used).

Containers for Reusable Sharps

Contaminated sharps that are reusable are to be placed immediately, or as soon as possible, after use into appropriate sharps containers. At this facility, the sharps containers are puncture resistant, are labeled with a biohazard label, and are leakproof. (Employers should list here where sharps containers are located as well as who has responsibility for removing sharps from containers and how often the containers will be checked to remove the sharps.)

Work-Area Restrictions

In work areas where there is a reasonable likelihood of exposure to blood or other potentially infectious materials, employees are not to eat, drink, apply cosmetics or lip balm, smoke, or handle contact lenses. Food and beverages are not to be kept in refrigerators, freezers, shelves, cabinets, or countertops or benchtops where blood or OPIMs are present.

Mouth pipetting/suctioning of blood or other potentially infectious materials is prohibited.

All procedures will be conducted in a manner that will minimize splashing, spraying, splattering, and generation of droplets of blood or OPIMs. Methods to accomplish this goal at this facility are:

_____

(list methods, such as covers on centrifuges or usage of dental dams if appropriate).

Specimens

Specimens of blood or other potentially infectious materials will be placed in a container that prevents leakage during the collection, handling, processing, storage, and transport of the specimens.

The container used for this purpose will be labeled or color coded in accordance with the requirements of the OSHA standard. (Employers should note that the standard provides for an exemption for specimens from the labeling/color-coding requirement of the standard provided that the facility uses universal precautions in the handling of all specimens and the containers are recognizable as container specimens. This exemption applies only while the specimens remain in the facility. If the employer chooses to use this exemption, then it should be stated here.)

Any specimens that could puncture a primary container will be placed within a puncture-resistant secondary container. (The employer should list here how this will be carried out, for example, which specimens, if any, could puncture a primary container, which containers can be used as secondary containers, and where the secondary containers are located at the facility.)

If outside contamination of the primary container occurs, the primary container shall be placed within a secondary container that prevents leakage during the handling, processing, storage, transport, or shipping of the specimen.

Contaminated Equipment

Equipment that has become contaminated with blood or other potentially infectious materials shall be examined before servicing or shipping and shall be decontaminated as necessary unless the decontamination of the equipment is not feasible. (Employers should list here any equipment that cannot be decontaminated before servicing or shipping.)

Personal Protective Equipment

All personal protective equipment used at this facility will be provided without cost to employees. Personal protective equipment will be chosen based on the anticipated exposure to blood or other potentially infectious materials. The protective equipment will be considered appropriate only if it does not permit blood or other potentially infectious materials to pass through or reach the employees' clothing, skin, eyes, mouth, or other mucous membranes under normal conditions of use and for the duration of time that the protective equipment will be used.

Protective clothing will be provided to employees in the following manner: (list how the clothing will be provided to employees, for example, who has responsibility for distribution, and also list which procedures would require the protective clothing and the type of protections required. This could also be listed as an appendix to this program. The employer could use a checklist as follows):

Personal Protective Equipment	Task
☐ Gloves	_____
☐ Lab coat	_____
☐ Face shield	_____
☐ Clinic jacket	_____
☐ Protective eyewear (with solid side shield)	_____
☐ Surgical gown	_____
☐ Shoe covers	_____
☐ Utility gloves	_____
☐ Examination gloves	_____
☐ Other (list other personal protective equipment)	_____

All personal protective equipment will be cleaned, laundered, and disposed of by the employer at no cost to employees. All repairs and replacements will be made by the employer at no cost to employees.

All garments that are penetrated by blood shall be removed immediately or as soon as feasible. All personal protective equipment will be removed before leaving the work area. The following protocol has been developed to facilitate leaving the equipment at the work area: _____ (list where employees are expected to place the personal protective equipment on leaving the work area, and other protocols).

Gloves shall be worn where it is reasonably anticipated that employees will have hand contact with blood, other potentially infectious materials, nonintact skin, and mucous membranes. Gloves will be available from (state location and/or person who will be responsible for distributing gloves). Gloves will be used for the following procedures: _____ (list procedures).

Disposable gloves used at the facility are not to be washed or decontaminated for reuse and are to be replaced as soon as practical when they become contaminated or as soon as feasible if they are torn or punctured or when their ability to function as a barrier is compromised. Utility gloves may be decontaminated for reuse provided that the integrity of the glove is not compromised. Utility gloves will be discarded if they are cracked, peeling, torn, punctured, or exhibit other signs of deterioration or when their ability to function as a barrier is compromised.

Masks in combination with eye protection devices, such as goggles or glasses with solid side shield or chin-length face shield, are required to be worn whenever splashes, spray, splatter, or droplets of blood or other potentially infectious materials may be generated and eye, nose, or mouth contamination can reasonably be anticipated. Situations at this facility that would require such protection are as follows:

_____.

The OSHA standard also requires appropriate protective clothing to be used, such as lab coats, gowns, aprons, clinic jackets, or similar outer garments. The following situations require that such protective clothing be worn: _____.

Housekeeping

This facility will be cleaned and decontaminated according to the following schedule: _____ (list area and time).

Decontamination will be accomplished by using the following materials: (list the materials to be used, such as bleach solutions or EPA-registered germicides). All contaminated work surfaces will be decontaminated after completion of procedures, immediately or as soon as feasible after any spill of blood or other potentially infectious materials, as well as at the end of the work shift if surfaces may have become contaminated since the last cleaning. (Employers should add any information concerning the use of protective coverings such as plastic wrap that keeps the surfaces free of contamination.)

All bins, pails, cans, and similar receptacles shall be inspected and decontaminated on a regularly scheduled basis (list frequency and by whom).

Any broken glassware that may be contaminated will not be picked up directly with the hands. The following procedures will be used: _____.

Labels

The following labeling method(s) is used in this facility:

EQUIPMENT TO BE LABELED	LABEL TYPE (size, color, etc.)
_____	_____
_____	_____

(**Name of responsible person or department**) will ensure that warning labels are affixed or red bags are used as required if regulated waste or contaminated equipment is brought into the facility. Employees are to notify _____ if they discover regulated waste containers, refrigerators containing blood or OPIMs, contaminated equipment, etc., without proper labels.

Regulated Waste Disposal

All contaminated sharps shall be discarded as soon as feasible in sharps containers located in the facility. Sharps containers are located in _____ (specify locations of sharps containers).

Regulated waste other than sharps shall be placed in appropriate containers. Such containers are located in _____ (specify locations of containers).

Laundry Procedures

Laundry contaminated with blood or other potentially infectious materials will be handled as little as possible. Such laundry will be placed in appropriately marked bags where it was used. Such laundry will not be sorted or rinsed in the area of use.

All employees who handle contaminated laundry will use personal protective equipment to prevent contact with blood or other potentially infectious materials.

Laundry at this facility will be cleaned at: _____ (specify location). [(Employers should note here if the laundry is being sent offsite. If the laundry is being sent offsite, then the laundry service accepting the laundry is to be notified, in accordance with section (d) of the standard.)]

Hepatitis B Vaccine

All employees who have been identified as having exposure to blood or other potentially infectious materials will be offered the hepatitis B vaccine at no cost to the employee. The vaccine will be offered within 10 working days of their initial assignment to work involving the potential for occupational exposure to blood or other potentially infectious materials unless the employee has previously had the vaccine or wishes to submit to antibody testing that shows the employee to have sufficient immunity.

Employees who decline the hepatitis B vaccine will sign a waiver that uses the wording in Appendix A of the OSHA standard.

Employees who initially decline the vaccine but who later wish to have it while still covered under standard may then have the vaccine provided at no cost. (Employers should list here who has responsibility for assuring that the vaccine is offered, the waivers are signed, etc. Also, the employer should list who will administer the vaccine.)

Documentation of refusal of the vaccination is kept at (**list location or person responsible for this record keeping**).

Vaccination will be provided by (**list health care professional who is responsible for this part of the plan**) at (**location**).

After hepatitis B vaccinations, the health care professional's written opinion will be limited to whether the employee requires the hepatitis vaccine and whether the vaccine was administered.

Postexposure Evaluation and Follow-up

When the employee incurs an exposure incident, it should be reported to: (**list who has responsibility to maintain records of exposure incident**).

All employees who incur an exposure incident will be offered postexposure evaluation and follow-up in accordance with the OSHA standard.

This follow-up will include the following:

- Documentation of the route of exposure and the circumstances related to the incident.
- If possible, the identification of the source individual and, if possible, the status of the source individual. The blood of the source individual will be tested (after consent is obtained) for HIV/HBV infectivity.
- Results of testing of the source individual will be made available to the exposed employee with the exposed employee informed about the applicable laws and regulations concerning disclosure of the identity and infectivity of the source individual. (Employers may need to modify this provision in accordance with applicable local laws on this subject. Modifications should be listed here.)
- The employee will be offered the option of having his or her blood collected for testing of the employee's HIV/HBV serological status. The blood sample will be preserved for up to 90 days to allow the employee to decide whether

the blood should be tested for HIV serological status; however, if the employee decides before that time that testing will or will not be conducted, then the appropriate action can be taken and the blood sample discarded.

- The employee will be offered postexposure prophylaxis in accordance with the current recommendations of the U.S. Public Health Service. These recommendations are currently as follows: (these recommendations may be listed as an appendix to the plan).
- The employee will be given appropriate counseling concerning precautions to take during the period after the exposure incident. The employee will also be given information on what potential illness to be alert for and to report any related experiences to appropriate personnel.

The following person(s) has been designated to assure that the policy outlined here is effectively carried out as well as to maintain records related to this policy:

_____

Interaction With Health Care Professionals

A written opinion shall be obtained from the health care professional who evaluates employees of this facility. Written opinions will be obtained in the following instances:

1. When the employee is sent to obtain the hepatitis B vaccine
2. Whenever the employee is sent to a health care professional after an exposure incident

Health care professionals shall be instructed to limit their opinions to:

1. Whether the hepatitis B vaccine is indicated and if the employee has received the vaccine, or for evaluation following an incident.
2. That the employee has been informed of the results of the evaluation.
3. That the employee has been told about any medical conditions resulting from exposure to blood or other potentially infectious materials. (Note that the written opinion to the employer is not to reference any personal medical information.)

Employee Training

All employees who have occupational exposure to bloodborne pathogens receive training conducted by (**name of responsible person or department**). (**Attach a brief description of their qualifications**.)

All employees who have occupational exposure to bloodborne pathogens receive training on the epidemiology, symptoms, and transmission of bloodborne pathogen diseases. In addition, the training program covers, at a minimum, the following elements:

1. A copy and explanation of the standard
2. An explanation of our ECP and how to obtain a copy
3. An explanation of methods to recognize tasks and other activities that may involve exposure to blood and OPIMs, including what constitutes an exposure incident
4. An explanation of the use and limitations of engineering controls, work practices, and PPE
5. An explanation of the types, uses, location, removal, handling, decontamination, and disposal of PPE
6. An explanation of the basis for PPE selection
7. Information on the hepatitis B vaccine, including information on its efficacy, safety, method of administration, the benefits of being vaccinated, and that the vaccine will be offered free of charge
8. Information on the appropriate actions to take and persons to contact in an emergency involving blood or OPIMs
9. An explanation of the procedure to follow if an exposure incident occurs, including the method of reporting the incident and the medical follow-up that will be made available
10. Information on the postexposure evaluation and follow-up that the employer is required to provide for the employee following an exposure incident
11. An explanation of the signs and labels and/or color coding required by the standard and used at this facility
12. An opportunity for interactive questions and answers with the person conducting the training session

Training materials for this facility are available at:

_____

_____

_____.

Record Keeping

Annual Review

The ECP shall be reviewed and updated at least annually and whenever necessary to reflect new or modified tasks and procedures which affect occupational exposure and to reflect new or revised employee positions with occupational exposure. The review and update of such plans shall also:

1. Reflect changes in technology that eliminate or reduce exposure to bloodborne pathogens
2. Document annually consideration and implementation of appropriate commercially available and effective safer medical devices designed to eliminate or minimize occupational exposure

Employee Input

The ECP identifies and documents the process by which the employer solicits input from nonmanagerial employees responsible for direct patient care who are potentially exposed to injuries from contaminated sharps in the identification, evaluation, and selection of effective engineering and work practice controls.

Sharps Injury Log

A sharps injury log is established, maintained, and consistently reviewed for recording of percutaneous injuries from contaminated sharps. The sharps injury log is maintained in such a way to ensure that information concerning the injured employee remains confidential.

The sharps injury log must contain, at a minimum, the following:

1. The type and brand of device involved in the incident
2. The department or work area where the exposure incident occurred

3. An explanation of how the incident occurred

Training Records

Training records are completed for each employee upon completion of training. These documents will be kept for at least three years at: (**name of responsible person or location of records**).

The training records include the following:
- The dates of the training sessions
- The contents or a summary of the training sessions
- The names and qualifications of persons conducting the training
- The names and job titles of all persons attending the training sessions

Employee training records are provided upon request to the employee or the employee's authorized representative within 15 working days. Such requests should be addressed to: (**name of responsible person or department**).

Medical Records

Medical records are maintained for each employee with occupational exposure in accordance with 29 CFR 1910.20, "Access to Employee Exposure and Medical Records."

(**Name of responsible person or department**) is responsible for maintenance of the required medical records. These **confidential** records are kept at: (**list location**) for at least the **duration of employment plus 30 years**.

Employee medical records are provided upon request of the employee or to anyone having written consent of the employee within 15 working days. Such requests should be sent to: (**name of responsible person or department and address**).

OSHA Record Keeping

An exposure incident is evaluated to determine if the case meets OSHA's Recordkeeping Requirements (29 CFR 1904). This determination and the recording activities are done by: (**name of responsible person or department**).

Tuberculosis

▶ Introduction

Why Is Tuberculosis Included in a Bloodborne Pathogens Manual?

This section contains information about tuberculosis (TB), an airborne disease. Since 1985, the incidence of TB in the general U.S. population has increased approximately 14%, reversing a 30-year downward trend. Recently, drug-resistant strains of *Mycobacterium tuberculosis (M tuberculosis)* have become a serious concern, and cases of multidrug-resistant (MDR) TB have occurred in 40 states. This overview of the risks of tuberculosis exposure (although it is not a bloodborne pathogen) has been added because many employees with occupational exposure to bloodborne pathogens may potentially have occupational exposure to persons with TB.

Nationwide, at least several hundred health care workers (HCWs) have become infected with TB and have required medical treatment after workplace exposure to TB. Twelve of these HCWs have died of TB. In general, persons who become infected with TB have approximately a 10% risk for developing TB in their lifetimes.

2005 Centers for Disease Control and Prevention TB Guidelines

OSHA has not released a standard specific to tuberculosis (as of this printing); however, the Centers for Disease Control and Prevention (CDC) has released the 2005 TB Guidelines for the protection of HCWs. OSHA believes the CDC's 2005 TB Guidelines reflect an industry recognition of the hazard as well as appropriate, widely recognized, and accepted standards of practice to be followed by employers in carrying out their responsibilities under the act.

The CDC is not a regulatory agency. The focus of the 2005 CDC TB Guidelines is to minimize the number of HCWs exposed to *M tuberculosis* while maintaining optimum care of patients with active infection with *M tuberculosis*. The guidelines can be found in the *Morbidity and Mortality Weekly Report*, vol. 54, December 30, 2005, No. RR-17, "Recommendations and Reports: Guidelines for Preventing the Transmission of *Mycobacterium tuberculosis* in Health-Care Facilities."

Occupational Safety and Health Act of 1970

OSHA is a regulatory agency. OSHA regulations are written to protect the employee from recognized hazards in the workplace. OSHA can and does enforce the worker protection by invoking the Occupational Safety and Health Act of 1970, or the General Duty Clause. The General Duty Clause (Public Law 91-596) states that "each employer shall furnish to each of his employees employment and a place of employment which are free from recognized hazards that are causing or are likely to cause death or serious physical harm to his employees: shall comply with occupational safety and health standards promulgated under this Act. Each employee shall comply with occupational safety and health standards and all rules, regulations, and orders issued pursuant to this Act which are applicable to his own actions and conduct."

Methods are available to minimize the hazards posed by employee exposure to TB. It is the employer's responsibility to see that these protections are in place and are readily available. It is your (the employee's) responsibility to use these protections.

Who Needs This Section?

Any employee who has potential for occupational exposure to *M tuberculosis* needs this section. The 2005 CDC TB Guidelines specify several potentially hazardous work settings:

- Health care facilities
- Long-term care facilities for older persons
- Homeless shelters
- Drug and treatment centers
- Correctional facilities

Health care facilities include inpatient settings (emergency departments, patient rooms), outpatient settings (medical offices, dialysis units), and nontraditional facility-based settings (EMS, home-based health care). The CDC also notes that TB patients might be encountered in other settings as well, such as laundry facilities, pharmacies, and law enforcement settings.

The following is a list of HCWs whose tasks may lead them to occupational exposure to *M tuberculosis*. The potential for occupational exposure is not limited to employees in these positions.

- Physicians
- Nurses
- Aides
- Home health care workers
- Dental workers
- Technicians
- Workers in laboratories and morgues
- Emergency medical service personnel
- Students
- Part-time personnel
- Temporary staff not employed by the health care facility
- Persons not directly involved with patient care, but who are potentially at risk for occupational exposure to *M tuberculosis* (eg, air ventilation system workers)

Meeting the General Duty Clause

The 2005 CDC TB Guidelines specify steps to be taken in order to minimize exposure to *M tuberculosis*. In order to ensure a safe working environment and meet the OSHA General Duty Clause requirements, employers should provide the following:

1. An assessment of the risk for transmission of *M tuberculosis* in the particular work setting
2. A protocol for the early identification of individuals with active TB
3. Training and information to ensure employee knowledge of the method of TB transmission, its signs and symptoms, medical surveillance and therapy, and site-specific protocols, including the purpose and proper use of controls (failure to provide respirator training is citable under OSHA's general industry standard on respirators)
4. Medical screening, including preplacement evaluation; administration and interpretation of Mantoux skin tests
5. Evaluation and management of workers with positive skin tests or a history of positive skin tests who are exhibiting symptoms of TB, including work restrictions for infectious employees
6. AFB (acid-fast bacilli) isolation rooms for suspected or confirmed infectious TB patients. These AFB isolation rooms and areas in which high-hazard procedures are performed should be single-patient rooms with special ventilation characteristics that are properly installed, maintained, and evaluated to reduce the potential for airborne exposure to *M tuberculosis*.
7. Institution of exposure controls specific to the workplace which include the following:
   - Administrative controls are policies and procedures to reduce the risk of employee exposure to infectious sources of *M tuberculosis*. An example is a protocol to ensure rapid detection of people who are likely to have an active case of TB.
   - Engineering controls attempt to design safety into the tools and workspace organization. An example is High Efficiency Particulate Air (HEPA) filtration systems.
   - Personal respiratory protective equipment is used by the employee to prevent exposure to potentially infectious air droplet nuclei, for example, a personal respirator.

► Tuberculosis (TB)

What Is Tuberculosis?

- *M tuberculosis* is the bacteria responsible for causing TB in humans.
- TB is a disease that primarily spreads from person to person through droplet nuclei suspended in the air.
- TB may cause disease in any organ of the body. The most commonly affected organ is the lung, which accounts for about 85% of all infection sites. Other sites may include lymph nodes, the central nervous system, kidneys, and the skeletal system.
- TB is a serious and often fatal disease if left untreated.
- Symptoms of TB include weight loss, weakness, fever, night sweats, coughing, chest pain, and coughing up blood.
- The prevalence of infection is much higher in the close contacts of TB patients than in the general population.
- There is a difference between TB infection (positive TB skin test) and TB disease.

Transmission

TB is spread from person to person in the form of droplet nuclei in the air. When a person with TB coughs, sings, or laughs, the droplet nuclei are released into the air. When uninfected people breathe in the droplet nuclei, they may become infected with TB.

For an employee to develop TB infection, he or she must have close contact to a sufficient number of air droplet nuclei. The employee's health is also considered as contributing to the susceptibility for TB infection and the possible development of TB disease. Among the medical risk factors for developing TB are diabetes, gastrectomy (removal of the stomach), long-term corticosteroid use, immunosuppressive therapy, cancers and other malignancies, and HIV infection.

Symptoms

Symptoms of TB also occur in people with more common diseases such as a cold or flu. The difference is that the symptoms of TB disease last longer than those of a cold or flu and must be treated with prescription antibiotics. The usual symptoms of TB disease include cough, production of sputum, weight loss, loss of appetite, weakness, fever, night sweats, malaise, fatigue, and, occasionally, chest pain. Hemoptysis, the coughing up of blood, may also occur, but usually not until after a person has had TB disease for some time.

Diagnosis

TB disease is diagnosed when there is a positive AFB sputum smear or when three successive early morning sputum specimens are cultured and there is growth of *M tuberculosis* from at least one culture. When extrapulmonary (not in the lungs) TB is being considered, it may also be diagnosed by culture techniques. The difference is that the specimen is cultured from the site where TB is considered as the cause of the infection.

► Prevention

The 2005 CDC TB Guidelines recommend a hierarchy of controls to minimize TB transmission. These strategies are used in combination to promote workplace safety and to provide the employee with maximum protection against occupational exposure to *M tuberculosis*. Under these guidelines, the control of TB is to be accomplished through the early identification, isolation, and treatment of persons with TB; the use of engineering and administrative procedures to reduce the risk of exposure; and through the use of respiratory protection. The CDC 2005 TB Guidelines also stress the importance of the following measures: (1) use of risk assessments for developing a written TB control plan (eg, incidence of TB in your community, number of patients with TB admitted to your facility), (2) TB screening programs for HCWs, (3) HCW training and education, and (4) evaluation of TB infection-control programs.

► TB Screening

Who Should Receive TB Screening?

According to the 2005 CDC TB Guidelines, HCWs are at increased risk for TB infection and should be provided with TB skin testing. This testing must be provided at no cost to employees at risk of exposure. The general population of the United States is thought to be at low risk for TB and should not be routinely tested.

Frequency of Testing

The frequency of testing is determined by the number of active cases of TB within a worksite of the facility. HCWs should receive TB skin testing before work in an area at increased risk for active cases of TB. A two-step TB skin testing process should be used (see What Is the Booster Effect?). Testing should be repeated each year or more frequently for an employee assigned to a high-risk worksite or after a known exposure to a person with active TB.

What Is the TB Skin Test?

The tuberculin skin test of choice is the Mantoux test, which uses an intradermal injection of purified protein derivative (PPD). There are three strengths of PPD available; intermediate-strength (five tuberculin units) PPD is the standard test material.

A skin test is done by injecting a very small amount of PPD just under the skin (usually the forearm is used). A small bleb (bump) will be raised. The bleb will disappear. The injection site is then checked for reaction by your clinician about 48 to 72 hours later. If you fail to have the injection site evaluated in 72 hours and no induration (swelling) is present, the tuberculin skin test will need to be repeated.

What Types of Reactions Occur?

Induration, the hard and bumpy swelling at the injection site, is used for determining a reaction to the PPD. Interpretation of results are best understood when the general health and risk of exposure to active TB cases are considered in the assessment. The injection site may also be red, but that does not determine a reaction to the PPD nor indicate a positive result. We recommend that the interpretation guidelines of the American Thoracic Society–CDC Advisory panel be used to assess the measured induration at the injection site.

What Does a Positive Result Mean?

A positive skin test means an infection with *M tuberculosis* has occurred, but does not prove TB disease. Referral for further medical evaluation is required to determine a diagnosis of TB disease. People found to

have TB disease must be provided effective treatments. These treatments would be provided to the employee by the employer if the illness was found to be work related.

Possible False-Positive Results

Close contacts of a person with TB disease who have had a negative reaction to the first skin test should be retested about 10 weeks after the last exposure to the person with TB disease. The delay between tests should allow enough time for the body's immune system to respond to an infection with *M tuberculosis*. A second test will result in a positive reaction at the injection site if an infection with *M tuberculosis* has occurred.

Contraindications to TB Screening

If you have tested positive to the TB skin test in the past, it is not recommended that you receive the test again. If you have had a vaccine called BCG (sometimes used in foreign countries), you should not have a TB skin test, since it will be positive.

Pregnancy does not exclude an HCW from being tested. Many pregnant workers have been tested for TB without documented harm to the fetus. You should consult with your doctor if you are pregnant and have any questions about receiving a TB skin test.

▶ Postexposure Reporting

What Determines an Occupational Exposure?

Occupational exposure to *M tuberculosis* is defined as employees working in one of the types of facilities whose workers have been identified by the CDC as having a higher incidence of TB than the general population, and whose employees have exposure defined as follows:

1. Potential exposure to the exhaled air of an individual with suspected or confirmed TB disease
2. Exposure to a high-hazard procedure performed on an individual with suspected or confirmed TB disease, which could generate potentially infectious airborne droplet nuclei

What Is the Booster Effect?

Sensitivity to the TB skin test may decrease over time, causing an initial skin test to be negative but at the same time stimulating or boosting the immune system's sensitivity to tuberculin, thereby producing a positive reaction the next time the test is given. When repeated skin testing is necessary, concern about the booster effect and the misinterpretation of skin test results can be avoided by using a two-step testing process. This is why your employer should require the two-step test as soon as you start employment. The two-step test helps to eliminate any confusion over whether an employee was infected at the worksite or was previously infected (see Record Keeping).

Postexposure Evaluation and Testing

Record Keeping

Records of employee exposure to TB, skin tests, and medical evaluations and treatment must be maintained by your employer.

Active tuberculosis disease is an illness that must be reported to public health officials. Every state has reporting requirements.

For OSHA Form 200 record-keeping purposes, both tuberculosis infections (positive TB skin test) and tuberculosis disease are recordable. A positive skin test for tuberculosis, even on initial testing (except preassignment screening), is recordable on the OSHA 200 log because of the presumption of work relatedness in these settings, unless there is clear documentation that an outside exposure occurred.

▶ Requirements

TB Exposure Control Plan

Employers having employees with exposure to TB shall establish a written exposure control plan designed to eliminate or minimize employee exposure. This plan involves the following:

- Schedule and method of implementation of the control plan
- PPD testing
- Respiratory protection
- Communication of hazards to employees
- Postexposure evaluation and follow-up
- Record keeping

Relationship to HIV

1. People infected with HIV and *M tuberculosis* are at a very high risk of developing active TB. Seven percent to 10% of persons infected with both TB and HIV will develop active disease each year.
2. Extrapulmonary TB (ie, outside the lungs) is more common in people with HIV infections.
3. Miliary TB (infection that has spread to other organs by the blood or lymph system) and lymphatic TB (infection of the lymphatic glands) are more common in HIV-infected persons.
4. The HIV epidemic is a major contributing factor to the recent increase in cases of active TB.

image credits

Chapter 1

Opener Courtesy of Kimberly Smith/CDC;
1-2 © LiquidLibrary.

Chapter 2

Opener © PhotoSpin, Inc./Alamy Images; 2-3 © Mikhail
Olykainen/ShutterStock, Inc.

Chapter 3

Opener © David E. Waid/ShutterStock, Inc.;
3-5 © Vadim Kozlovsky/ShutterStock, Inc.;
3-7 Courtesy of Kimberly Smith and Christine
Ford/CDC; 3-8 Courtesy of Kimberly Smith/CDC;
3-13 © Wayne Johnson/ShutterStock, Inc.

Chapter 4

Opener © joe outland/Alamy Images; 4-2 Courtesy of
Jim Gathany/CDC.

Chapter 5

Opener © Graca Victoria/ShutterStock, Inc.

Unless otherwise indicated, photographs are under
copyright of Jones and Bartlett Publishers, Inc., courtesy
of MIEMSS, or the American Academy of Orthopaedic
Surgeons.